READER F

"Wow! What an amazing writer *and* singer you are. Your writing captivated me. It was so easy to understand. I could feel the emotion!"

— *Don Tolman, The Wholefood Medicine Man*

"Alicia Blickfeldt's new memoir *They Said I Would Die* carries the reader along through a fascinating, emotional journey of sheer will, faith, and fortitude as she faces off against the unrelenting devils that have plagued humanity since the beginning of time—fear, discouragement, physical weakness and pain. Through it all, Alicia guides the reader along through the maze of doubt and despair into the light that awaits all honest seekers of truth. Come along and experience with Alicia the quest for victory as she battles for her very life and, perhaps more importantly, her very soul . . . ."

— *Shanna Francis, newspaper editor and publisher*

"This is a true story of holistic healing, spirituality and faith. Alicia shows us how food and prayer are medicines that can be utilized to heal, by enhancing our own body's ability to heal itself. She shows how our western world of medicine has become corrupt always looking for monetary gain by pushing radical chemical treatments which poison the body while attempting to perhaps cure it."

— *Gina Gonzalez, Realtor, Business Owner, MIT graduate*

"I just finished your book! I loved reading your entire story and seeing the progression of your faith. It has given me reflection on my own life and how I handle the challenges that come my way."

— *Melanie Shaw, wife, mother and friend*

"I have been avoiding medical treatment for two years. This book has given me hope, and that it is okay to follow my gut feelings and spiritual inspiration!"

— *Valorie Chapman, holistic energy worker*

"Alicia tells a clear and honest story that will assist the reader in developing a desire to take personal control of his or her health (physically, mentally, and spiritually) and learn of alternative methods of healing."

— *Annette Slade, lover of all natural foods*

WHERE TO FIND ALICIA BLICKFELDT

FACEBOOK

REVERBNATION

TWITTER

SOUNDCLOUD

INSTAGRAM

&

ON YOUTUBE, YOU WILL FIND AN ARTISTIC INTERPRETATION OF

THE JOURNEY DESCRIBED IN THIS BOOK. IT IS CALLED

PIE JESU, THE PROCESS OF REDEMPTION

#FILLINGTHEWORLDWITHLIGHT

They Said

I WOULD

DIE

❦

A journey to self-healing

They Said

I WOULD

DIE

A journey to self-healing

ALICIA BLICKFELDT

ISBN-13: 978-1539018674
ISBN-10: 1539018679

Published by Alicia Blickfeldt, aliciablickfeldt@gmail.com

FIRST EDITION

Blickfeldt, Alicia
They said I would die, a journey to self-healing / Alicia Blickfeldt

Cover design by Alicia Blickfeldt
Cover design © 2017 by Alicia Blickfeldt

Printed in the United States of America.

ACKNOWLEDGEMENTS

Thank you to the many hands that made the work of completing this book light. Bless you for your countless hours of edits, refinements and expressions of encouragement. You have made my life more meaningful for being a part of this project! May the Master of us all fill your lives with joy.

Shanna Francis, Editor

RayDean Hill, Editor

Annette Slade, Editor

Gina Gonzalez, Editor

Greg Madson, Editor

Paul Cactus Jack La Marr, Editor

Valorie Chapman, Reader

Diana Ludwig, Reader

Mechelle R. McDermott, Reader

In Gratitude

To Jesus the Christ,
for unwearyingly teaching me how to heal.

To Mike, without whom I might have faltered and taken a different road,
and whose calm spirit continually encouraged me.

To Mom, who sat by my bed,
fed me every day
and saw to my every need. Bless you.

To Dad, who let me have my mother
for five very *long* weeks.

To Melanie Shaw who heard an inspired thought
and delivered it to me,
which led to the writing of this book.

To numerous friends and editors
whose critical input and assistance
were crucial to this project.

CONTENTS

CONTENTS

INTRODUCTION

Self-healing. It is a bit of a buzz word these days. Some say the idea is good, others think it is crazy. Admittedly, I have not always been one of those who thought it was necessarily good, but life, as we know, has a tendency to teach us lessons we may not really wish to learn, even though they are nearly always for our benefit.

Such was my lesson, or lessons, as it were. I have become an expert in the act of healing myself. It has not been an easy road. Nor do I presume to suggest it is the road you ought to take. I am, however, an advocate of self-healing—it is what I believe in. What I feel and have experienced has taught me that my body *can* heal itself—*if* I am willing to pay the price and, in my case, willing to humble myself and ask God for His help.

A number of years ago I had a modest interest in health and nutrition that, like most things, was adhered to only when there were no obvious temptations nearby. My interest swung from meaninglessness—if I were hungry—to self-righteous "knowledge," if I were not. Unfortunately, I talked the talk but failed to diligently walk the walk.

I had a valid excuse—my body felt fit and I was always thin! So that meant I was healthy—right? I never could understand going to the doctor just for a check-up. I adhere to the old adage, "If it ain't broke, don't fix it." Besides, becoming sick was never going to happen to me. I was confident and full of life and vitality. Never had the idea crossed my mind that I could become seriously ill. Then, one unexpected and unforeseen day, everything changed. Dis-ease did enter my world.

Devastation was the pervading emotion that resonated through me during those first few months after discovering how ill I really was. But through miracle after miracle, each step I took drew me closer to understanding the truth about how the human body functions, and how it responds to positive stimulus. Just like a baby who sees and is attracted to a shiny object, I just kept crawling closer and closer towards self-healing until I could almost touch it. And then, at the end of the journey, I grabbed hold with all my might and never looked back.

My hope is that my experience will inspire you; perhaps it will even open your mind to greater possibilities. Even if it just seems like a nice story, for me, it was the journey of a lifetime along a path that had more dips and weaves than a thrilling ride at an amusement park.

But more than just a nice story, this book is a book of hope—and of joy! It provides a different perspective of, not only health, but life. And while it is not for me to decide which path is right for you, if you grasp and apply the concepts from my experience, it may just change the way you look and care for yourself in every imaginable way.

Let the journey begin!

Chapter One

IMAGINING MY DEATH

Denial. I was in immediate denial. A short blast of forced air escaped my lips in defiance as I recoiled like a mimosa plant, disallowing the possibility of the lump.

It worked for a minute, but now that I was cognizant of *"its"* presence, the "what ifs" took over, budding into a vapor that seemed to leach into every crevice of my soul.

The sun shone brightly that morning as I lifted my eyes to the mirror in front of me. "What could it be?" I thought to myself. I was the picture of health, I thought, so I was perplexed beyond imagination. "Surely it couldn't be—no!" I stopped myself short of actually venturing over the line to worst-case scenarios. For the next several minutes I methodically worked to squelch the obtrusive opinions one by one, countering with my own deliberate comments.

"I am healthy. My body heals itself each and every day," I said in silence.

What I was seeing on the outside of my body was mirrored by what I felt so profoundly on the inside—terror. I continued to mentally speak what I wanted to be my reality.

It helped calm me a bit. I leaned against the bathroom counter using both hands to brace myself. "I am healthy. I am strong," I whispered, and then my resolve began to waver. "What if this is serious? What if you have...." I stopped myself again as my chin began shaking violently.

Breaking the visual hold I had on myself, I tried not to let the tears drop from my eyes. Too late, they fell anyway: two, three, four splatters hitting the white porcelain of the sink.

Squeezing the edge of the counter, I drew in an awful breath grappling to control my emotions. "I am healthy," I said loudly enough to hear, but softly enough not to wake my husband in the next room. The conviction grew in my voice. "My body is in perfect working order."

It may seem a strange reaction to my discovery, but for several years previously I had been immersed in a self-driven, self-improvement, mentoring program. I had learned to regulate my thoughts, manifesting a multitude of positive things into my life. I had learned that everything was more blissful, productive and purpose-driven when I had a positive mindset.

When these new and unsolicited emotions attacked my now highly-trained, optimistic thought process, I instinctively fought back to not let my feelings get the best of me.

I went for months and told no one about the lump—not my parents, not my husband Mike—and not even God. Religion was a huge part of my life. It guided my thoughts and actions and was the force for good in my life. But here I was, hiding from the One who had the answers. I could not bring myself to discuss the topic with Him, so I left my fears out of my prayers, attempting to lessen the potential and hoping it was just something simple. I rationalized that if I thought positively enough, it would go away, and I held on to that hope.

It was not easy hiding it from everyone. At the most inopportune occasions, emotion would swing in, threatening to blow my cover. Many more times than I can count, I found myself heading for the bathroom, where I knew there would be an ample supply of toilet paper to dry my eyes.

Even more aggravating was the embarrassment I felt for even developing a lump in the first place. I blamed myself for it. Each time I allowed myself to be open to the options, I would sink into dark places and start listening to the never-ending barrage of loud voices in my head.

I would sometimes think about visiting a doctor, where I could get some sort of medical explanation. There was obviously no outside pressure to do so; I was the only one who knew. But if I committed to an appointment, that would be like admitting there was something wrong.

Not only was I frightened by the thought of what the lump really was, I had an issue with Westernized medical practices. In addition, we did not have health insurance. I used that as an excuse to not go.

In all honesty, the bottom line was that I was terrified about turning my power over to someone I did not know or trust, and who could potentially manipulate me into taking actions that I would normally never even consider. Maybe I was a little too independent, but fear held me in that place of limbo for a long time. Maybe it was an unseen blessing that I was unaware of at the time; so, I waited. And since I had chosen not to tell anyone about it, I was alone.

Over time, I got very good at not looking at the possibilities. From time to time they would rear up, but typically I would just ignore them. I became aware of just how powerful my mind was and how much domination I actually had over my own brainwaves. Somehow that gave me a sense of empowerment. My life smoothed out for the most part and I moved forward without giving too much consideration to the lump. Besides, it was nothing anyway.

However, one morning, I became aware of the gentle nudging of heaven, which was coaxing me to at least tell Mike. The idea petrified me. I was deeply concerned about Mike's reaction.

I do not know if the sun was shining that day or not. To me everything was grey and murky. I was far too wrapped up in the idea of breaking the news to Mike, and it covered me with heaviness and weighed on me greatly. As I thought about what I would say, it was as if a shadow passed in front of me; I was unsettled. I blinked hard, took in another breath and stood erect, gathering the necessary courage. "Okay, it's time," I thought to myself.

I stood straight, turned, and then stepped over the threshold that led into our bedroom. Mike was sitting on the edge of the bed. I hesitated slightly, then blurted out, "I have something I need to talk to you about."

Chapter Two

ADMISSIONS TO GOD

My words came out a bit louder than I had intended and it startled Mike. His head came up sharply and met my gaze. We had been married for 11 years, and he had learned that when I used that tone, he had better listen. Mike was an observer, maybe not of silly things like shoes or new hairdos, but he was completely keyed into my emotions and the nuances that accompanied occasions such as this. I had always appreciated that quality in him.

There is no doubt he saw the tightness of my lips. He stood swiftly, squared his shoulders, then took a couple of steps closer to me, his rich blue eyes intensifying as he examined the subtleties on my face.

My heart started to pound, and then I blurted, "I found a lump in my breast."

I probably should have found a gentler way to deliver the information, but it was all I could do to just formulate the words in the first place and then speak them into existence. Inside I felt a shudder, but managed to keep it hidden so Mike would not see it. His shoulders dropped ever so slightly and his cheek flinched just a little, telling me everything I needed to know. He was frightened. It alarmed me to see it.

Then he said, "Crap."

I felt the energy drain from my legs. I thought I might faint. In my chest the pounding became audible, as my breath grew shallow and quick. Every hair on my goose-bumped skin stood on end, filling me with the fear that I had worked so hard to bury. The shift in the room was palpable. I tightened inside and my stomach turned, the bile burning as it climbed up my esophagus.

I expected Mike was thinking the worst, and the gravity of it hit me like a brick. My head began to hurt and the thrashing of my heart expanded to my skull, banging loudly against the inside of my eardrums. Crimson patches were surfacing on the skin of my upper chest and neck, disclosing my anxiety. I hoped that he would not notice it in the dimly lit room because I did not want him to see how frightened I was becoming. I commanded my respiratory system to breathe regularly in an effort to still my soul, but it was no use.

Mike had not taken his eyes off me. I prayed he would not hear the hammering of my heart that I was so keenly aware of. I tried to hide my feelings from him, but he saw it. Terror mounted behind my eyes at his subtle but evident reaction, and I could feel myself slipping away, withdrawing into a shadowy cerebral hole.

Everything that happened over the next few minutes blurred as I became unaware of my surroundings. If Mike were talking, I did not hear it. I had retreated to somewhere empty and cold, where ugly phrases were bombarding me.

"What if it is *cancer*?"

There, I had actually entertained the word "cancer." The thought made me cringe. "What if I die?"

I let the axiom settle in on me, mentally weighing down as if sandbags had just been placed on each of my shoulders. Death. I wondered what that might look like. The implications were huge.

As my mind reeled out of control, one of the first unwelcome notions that crossed it was, "I wonder if Mike will marry someone else?" The thought burned like a hot poker stirring every thought together like a red-hot bed of coals. I felt faint. I could almost feel the steam rising from the top of my skull.

"Who would he marry?" In an instant I thought of Sarah. She was not single. At least not yet. Her abusive marriage had always disturbed me. I secretly wondered how close to divorce she might be and if she would even entertain the thought of marrying again. She was stunningly beautiful, talented on multiple fronts, spiritually in tune, and obviously very resilient to have such wonderful qualities under the duress of her life. Despite years of mental abuse, she was a really wonderful woman. As strange as it was, I entertained the idea that she would be an amazing companion for Mike. The fact the idea was developing into such a vision in my mind's eye did not set that well with me, but the images kept coming anyway.

As my brain slipped into overload, I became catatonic, staring blankly through the room and disappearing into my own dark reality. All I could see was Sarah moving into my role. She washed my dishes, she laughed at Mike's jokes, and she cuddled with him on the couch. Pictures slammed me relentlessly. He touched her hair as he walked through the room. She breathed in the subtle scent of aftershave on his neck in the glow of the fireplace. He squeezed her hand as they walked outdoors on a cool winter evening. So many thoughts. It was staggering.

I was frozen in place but became aware that my knees were tightly locked. The room began to spin. I would certainly faint if I did not disengage and allow the blood to flow. My legs were not responding. The onslaught in my head grew louder, drawing my attention back.

"What about the kids? What about their lives? I would miss it all! And they would miss me!" My stomach started rolling as another image of Sarah took over. I felt as if I had just jumped off a 40-foot cliff.

A flicker of reason flashed in me and I screamed in my own brain, "Stop!" A slight squeak may have slipped out, alerting Mike to the severity of where I was, but I did not move. I just stood stiff, wallowing in it as it played out in full-blown vivid images of a whole other life for him. I wanted to cry. I wanted to run, but my body was held in place by pictures of another time and place, and a life without me in it. It scrolled before my eyes like a movie.

The logistics of the scenario happened in only a split second. I visibly shivered and the next thing I knew, Mike's arms were wrapping around me, snapping me out of my vision just in time to catch me from falling. I bit my lip in an effort to squash the ache that was crushing my heart. My knees wobbled and the blood rushed to my brain, making me dizzy. The sadness completely enveloped me, but Mike's grasp held me firm as warmness gathered everywhere around, slowly drawing me back to reality.

"I love you," he said. "No matter what." The inflection in his voice was deep and sincere.

The energy of his words saturated my heart. Slowly, the pain began to lift out of my body, the sorrow began melting away, and the love I had come to know so solidly from him pierced my chest.

He pulled back and looked at me, trying to encourage me with a smile.

I gathered my nerve, attempting to recover from the earlier images of him with Sarah. I chose to focus on him, right there and then. I could feel the love he was intentionally transferring to me. It was steady, slowing my heartbeat. I looked into his eyes and knew he adored me, no one else.

It was as though Mike's love for me was being delivered as an electrical current, recharging my nearly empty battery. A single tear slipped from the left corner of my eye, dropping straight to the floor with a soft thud.

Finding my voice again I whispered, "Maybe it's just a cyst." It sounded tenuous and fragile, a flagrant deflection. I wanted to believe it and was trying to convince myself, as much as Mike, that the lump was nothing. I wanted it to be nothing. It *had* to be nothing.

After a few minutes of steeping in his tenderness, I felt better and heard myself start a rather drawn out, emotionally disconnected conversation about cysts. I went on and on about something I had read on the Internet, and something I had watched on a television show regarding them. My fingertips were numb from my constant arm flailing as I described it, and my eyes darted back and forth in an attempt to avoid eye contact. When I finally finished talking, Mike just said, "Huh. Maybe it is."

Whether or not he believed me, it was that smidgen of optimism that dangled like a carrot on a string in front of us. I shifted my attitude completely to that vein of thought. I would believe it into actuality! It was a cyst and everything would be okay!

~

Over the next few weeks the Internet became my go-to-girl. I would sit down and unearth information about cysts. It was informative, and helped stabilize the self-diagnosis I was clinging to. I fed off of the symptoms I learned about, and in my mind they were exactly the same as I was experiencing. It was a blatant attempt to create a truth I needed to be real.

I became rather proud of myself for seeking and finding answers that felt good to me. These positive emotions created a bubble that I was okay with living in, so I continued to feed myself with this line of thought.

There were days, however, when the underlying possibilities skated in and filled me with misgiving and question. On occasion, when Mike was not at home, I let my mind wander to the possibility of cancer. It always turned into something dark and depressing.

I would become disheartened and sullen as my mind fluctuated between my desired trust in God and His wisdom for my life, whatever that was to be, and my reoccurring fears. Instead of trusting, often I knowingly let the fears rule. I entertained them like an old friend. I invited them in and offered them a seat on my couch. I allowed those visits, sometimes for hours. Afterward I felt as though I had wallowed back and forth like a pig in a mud hole.

I thought about cancer and the disfiguring surgery that could mar my body for life. I thought about losing my hair and the humiliation I would feel. I thought about death and the life of my husband without me.

Those were gloomy days, exposing my lack of faith. That hurt more than all of the other thoughts combined.

After telling Mike about the lump, I broke down and told Heavenly Father, too. As I dropped to my knees and began pouring out my heart, I began to realize just how much He loved me. Without delay, my heart filled with tenderness and peace, and a sense settled in that everything would be all right, regardless of the outcome. Though it was hard for me to come to grips with the idea that death could be the end result, I was comforted by the understanding that God was fully aware of what was happening in my life.

Impressions came, revealing to me that I needed to prepare for what was to be—both in mind and body. Even though I prayed daily, I suddenly felt a deeper sense of urgency to get on my knees more frequently and up the ante on my faith, and to connect with all things spiritual. It brought peace and tranquility, but I still felt no urgency to rush to a doctor or clinic, so I postponed any medical visits.

Winter came. Christmas and New Year's flew by in a flurry of white. Then finally, after nine months of considerations and prayer, I decided to see a physician and, at least, get an idea of what the lump was. Oddly, I cannot say that I ever felt a strong spiritual notion to go, it just became something I decided to do. I found myself picking up the phone one day and making a call to the doctor. That was my first mistake, or so I thought for a long time.

For most of my life, I had never really been the type to visit doctors. In fact, it had been years since I had sought medical help. As I picked up my phone to make the call, my palms became moist and my heart began pounding. That should have been a clue that I was doing the "wrong thing." I could feel myself getting more and more anxious, even a little hostile, but with my current frame of reference and ignorance of the facts, I could not see another way of identifying the lump. In fact, I felt perplexed that I even needed to know what it was. But there I was, dialing. I heard myself confirm an appointment then hang up.

Confusion filled my mind and I disregarded what I would later come to believe was a spiritual warning. It was that moment when I felt as though I were giving up my will and handing it over to someone else. That impression would come back to haunt me time and time again.

I was petrified at the prospect of being thrown into the medical world. It was foreign and frightening to me. I had witnessed far too many medical outcomes that were not good. To me, there was zero positivity attached to a cancer diagnosis and the customary treatment options. In the media, cancer had been blown into something surreal and dreamlike, even nightmarish. If I participated in "the system," as I named it, it meant I might be intimidated into what I saw as an excessive over-prescribed, too-quick-to-suggest-surgery, experiment-with-human-life-for-money driven industry.

The only comfort I felt was that the abnormality in my breast had not changed since the day of my discovery. I had Mike check it from time to time in case my mental measurements were skewed by my familiarity with the growth. But even he detected no noticeable changes, which gave me confidence. This nine-month observation was the base line for everything that happened afterward.

Chapter Three

MARK OF THE BEAST

My plan was simple; I would go to the clinic and submit myself to an ultrasound. Based on what I had read online, it could be done without radiation and side effects. It sounded like a good idea at the time, but I had not truly considered the repercussions.

When I went into the clinic on the prearranged day, I felt fairly self-assured, but as the short, brown-haired nurse showed me to the examination room, a heavy sensation fell over me. She handed me a thin blue gown, and asked that I change into it. My thought of escaping vaporized. It was as though God was nudging me one last time. Justification kicked in. *"I'm already here. Maybe they'll have an answer."* I ignored the nudge and began disrobing.

A few minutes later, there was a knock on the door, followed by a female voice asking to come in. A woman, as tall as I am, with long blonde hair clipped back on the sides and pulled into an elastic band in the back, came in. She smiled, said her name was Lindsay, and proceeded to explain what would happen with the test, and then asked if I would sit on the examination table.

"Here we go." My brow furrowed. Pulsations of fear and anger expanded and contracted within me. I was angry that I had willingly placed myself into "the system."

Lindsay attempted to make me feel more comfortable as she helped me lay back on the table and adjusted my position. I saw a flash in her eyes as she uncovered my skin. The shock was written all over her face as she saw the obvious lump in my breast. I knew it and I was certain she knew it now, too. Then she explained that "he" would be in shortly. I squirmed. Why did it have to be a "he"? She covered me again and excused herself. Just before stepping out, she dimmed the lights in the room so the screen on the ultrasound monitor could easily be seen. It would have been comforting if I had not felt so vulnerable.

Four or five minutes passed, and I realized I was getting more nervous. Suddenly, there was a knock on the door. The technician came in, followed by a different nurse I did not recognize. His nametag read Caleb. He was friendly and efficient, and irritatingly young. He had short-cropped hair and pale eyes. He explained what he was about to do as he prepared the hand piece of the scanner with jelly. I bit my lip and closed my eyes. Seconds later I could feel my gown being moved aside and the scanner touching my skin. Promptly I grew hot with embarrassment. I wanted to shove him away and cover my body. Instead, I took in a slow deep breath. It was so controlled that Caleb likely did not even notice.

As he studied the black and white video screen, I turned so that I could see as well. Surprisingly, a large dark area showed. Then Caleb began speaking, describing what he was seeing and marking the size with a series of clicks. His speech grew loud as he started speaking. Panic seized me as he said that I needed to have multiple tests done today.

The tension in the room began to increase, and the fear I had dealt with for all those months pressed on me until I felt I would pass out from lack of oxygen.

Caleb finished, turned away and said something to the nurse—just long enough for me to sit up and awkwardly pull the gown tightly across my body. I was visibly shaking. A profound blackness seeped into the depths of my spirit. Feelings of confusion charged into me like an ocean wave, knocking my emotions back and forth from anger to dread, and back to anger again. He turned, speaking directly at me in that loud voice. I swear it went up in pitch.

Fear rose within me, the likes of which I had rarely experienced. I could not put together a cohesive thought. All I could do was listen to Caleb's words. My body felt rigid as I stared in his direction while a myriad of invisible voices screamed at me. Then, inexplicably, I heard myself agreeing to Caleb's suggestion for further tests. That was my second "mistake."

Dazed and completely out of my normal discipline, I submitted to their requests. For the next few hours I acquiesced to two mammograms, an x-ray, and a biopsy where Caleb not only withdrew tissue samples, but implanted a small titanium clip into my breast without asking.

As he inserted the clip, Caleb explained, "It's what we do to mark the spot for future images." He sounded almost jovial, as if he thought he was doing me some huge favor.

I blinked hard and stared in silence as coherency kicked in, "What did you just do? *You didn't even ask*! How dare you!" But none of these inner thoughts were coming out verbally. I was furious. I wanted to punch Caleb in the mouth and get out. But nothing moved and nothing escaped my lips. Sitting there motionless, I began to feel like a child who had been sent to the corner to face the wall.

Feeling slowly began to come back to my body and the anger began bubbling its way to the surface, so I breathed in and held my breath. Very distinct words were forming. Before they had a chance to explode into the room, I swallowed and bit my cheek, forcing them into silent obedience. I felt nauseous.

The potential ramifications of the clip "marking" me were all I could think about. What would any health insurance company say about that in the future, now that I was labelled a high risk patient? Premiums would skyrocket. A fleeting thought regarding the mark of the beast from the Bible came to me. This was not my hand or my forehead as is stated in Revelations, but it was an unwelcomed mark nonetheless. The worst effect from Caleb's careless and thoughtless action did not unveil itself to me until a few months later.

After Caleb left I sat silently. In the darkness of my heart, I vowed to never allow my agency to be revoked again. I dug a deep hole and planted a seed of insurrection.

Chapter Four

IT'S YOUR BODY

Marked by the clip, my anger toward Caleb remained and it took nearly the entire two-week period waiting for the test results to get through it.

Mike patiently listened as I blamed myself for all of it. I collapsed into a rueful heap on the floor. There was not much to be said, but Mike picked me up, put his arms around me and said, "It's going to be okay." I was grateful for his remark, but doubt still surfaced.

Mike was able to get a few hours off work and met me in the clinic parking lot to receive the results of the tests. It was late afternoon on a freezing winter day. The skies were cloudy and grey, and the air was interspersed with ice crystals. I rubbed my hands together and trembled as we entered the building. We were only seated there for a few minutes when my name was called.

Overall, I felt upbeat. I was convinced that it was a cyst for I spent more time than before studying it. We were led to a room that smelled like chemicals, making me a little woozy. My feelings of optimism wavered as the memories of my last visit moved in and landed squarely in front of me. I concentrated in an attempt to breathe rhythmically, praying to remain calm.

There was a knock on the door and the doctor came in. I was really beginning to hate that sound. It was growing to mean something unpleasant.

The doctor was tall and slightly heavy for her frame. She wore scrubs and a pair of crocs on her feet. Her long, frizzy, salt-and-pepper hair hung to the middle of her back and was pulled into a thick, somewhat unmanaged ponytail.

She looked a bit like a product of the '70s. In her hand was a manila file with my name printed across the top edge. She shook our hands in turn and introduced herself without smiling.

"Hello. I'm Dr. Calder," she pronounced with a flat and detached voice. Then she sat on a small black stool and scooted it forward into a position where she was sitting directly in front of me. She looked up with a stare that pierced me to the core, and suddenly my heart began to pound as if I were sitting in the principal's office for some high school offense.

Without much more than the introductory "hello," Dr. Calder announced, "You have cancer," delivering the verdict blankly and without emotion.

"What? Did you just say… no, it couldn't be. It is? It can't be. You need to rerun the tests because it's only a cyst," I said under my breath, until the realization settled in. "It's cancer? I'm going to…no…focus… it's going to be fine. It's going to be fine!"

I stared in disbelief, wondering if I had really heard her right. As the realization of her comments sunk in, I felt a look spread across my face that was nothing less than dumbfounded bewilderment. My face grew hot and I could feel my skin flushing with red blotches again. The walls began to close in and my entire body heated up as if it were suddenly 150 degrees.

Cancer. The word bounced around in my head like a huge boulder, smashing and tumbling down an imaginary embankment, looking for a solid place to land, damaging everything in its path and crushing me on its way by. That was it. *I have cancer.*

For a second time in that building, I sat immobile and taut as I tried to regain control of my mind and body. It was like a nightmarish replay of my last visit, and I could not move.

Dr. Calder stared, almost as if she were waiting for me to react. But I did not. I just stared back at her. I could feel the sweat beading up under the hair at the nape of my neck.

The facts had been presented—it was cancer—nothing more, nothing less. For a time I felt the crushing weight of the boulder. It had stopped rolling and had landed evenly between my shoulder blades. There was no pain, no terror, nothing, only a heavy numbness.

The doctor looked at me for what seemed like five minutes, waiting, but all that happened was an uncomfortable silence. Her comments hung in the air as though she had screamed it from the top of the chasm where the boulder had fallen from, echoing over and over.

Since I chose not to speak, she looked down at her chart and began delivering more information: the size of the tumor, what stage it was at, and where she thought I ought to go from here. It amazed me how easily she suggested the things she believed I should do—chemotherapy, radiation, surgery—as if it were a walk in the park. I watched her without really absorbing the material, disconcerted by the callous presentation.

My senses began returning and I turned to look at Mike, his mouth was open slightly and his eyes were glassed over. I could see with clarity that he was as baffled as I was. His eyes were locked on Dr. Calder, who was still droning on and flipping pages back and forth.

I glanced back toward the doctor, who had finally stopped talking, and I spoke, "Well, that was unexpected," I said in a tone that was so smooth and buttery that it almost tasted sweet in my mouth. It startled me and drew me inward as I began to process.

I stared; she was obviously talking again but nothing was getting in. I had completely blocked her out and was in my own world, trying to understand the inferences of her announcement. Then her voice trailed off and I came to an awareness that she had taken our silence as her cue to step out.

When the door was closed completely I turned and looked at Mike. He was stationary and emotionless, vacantly looking at the ramifications of the announcement as if someone had spread them out onto the floor in front of him. I breathed deeply, gathering courage to ask him a question and a little fearful of what his answer might be.

In a voice that sounded oddly sturdy I asked, "Do I have to do anything she just said?"

He turned and lifted his head to latch onto my gaze, and then he spoke. It was so far from what I expected him to say, that my mouth gaped open. His eyes intensified as they bore into mine, firmly fastening onto my consciousness. Then in a tone I had never heard from him before, he stated, "No. It's your body; you can do whatever you want."

It was a completely arbitrary comment, and one that most people would think was insane. To me it was flawless. Mike had just handed me a gift. The freedom to choose. He could have cried or begged, or pressed me into following the doctor's recommendations. Instead, he gave it to me to decide. That placed my love for him on a level I never saw coming. And it showed me that his love for me had no conditions.

The emotion I had been stifling erupted, but it was no longer fear, it was love. I think I even giggled. I stepped off the exam table just as Mike stood from the chair, scooping me into his arms. Wrapping myself into his embrace, I clung securely to his neck and thanked him for saying what he had. A few tears slipped from the edges of my eyes. Somehow, I knew everything would work out and I was certain that regardless of where this road was about to take us, Mike would be there—no matter what my decision ended up being.

"It's going to be okay," Mike whispered near my ear.

"Yes," I agreed quietly, "somehow it's going to work out."

Just then a strange energy seeped into my soul and for the moment I was filled with warmth and a sense of calm. It was like God was sending me a personal message of hope. I had just been delivered the gravest of sentences and yet I was at peace.

"Did you feel that?" I asked Mike, not daring to move.

"Yes," he responded in pleasant tones, "I did. The Lord loves you, Alicia. I think He wants you to know that."

I knew it. Warmth and tenderness had laced itself deep into my essence, if only for a fleeting moment. God was aware, and He would be there for me, too.

Unbeknownst to Mike, his words, and those heavenly feelings, had just given me the courage to take a huge step away from the doctor's suggestions. It sealed in me a powerful desire to explore a holistic approach to the problem.

Mike's phrase wafted through my thoughts again, "It's your body. . . ."

In a very literal sense, Mike had just saved my life. His words changed the course of everything I did from that day forward. But just as with everything, there had to be an opposing reaction.

Just as clearly as I had felt the spirit of Christ just minutes before, the balance in the room altered and Satan, who had been waiting in the wings, stepped in. Suddenly I was filled with hesitation. It baffled me that I felt that way at all since seconds before I knew my course. But there it was: confusion.

My resolve shook and then an outpouring of abuses in the form of negative self-talk began. I felt as though I were standing on the center of a seesaw that had suddenly fallen on one side. As soon as I became aware of his scheme, the stubbornness in me swelled and I was angry, an emotion I was glad to embrace just then. I dug my heels in, forcing the balance back to center.

Defiantly, the seeds of insurrection I had planted a few weeks earlier after my appointment with Caleb, popped open wide, stretching down and pushing the cold, dark soil away, sinking deep into my core where they began to take root. And even though I was scared and a bit tenuous about the direction I wanted to go, I recommitted to the plan that was forming within me. I did not know it then, but this would be just a tiny example of the emotional wave I was set upon.

Chapter Five

HE SLIPS IN WHEN YOU LEAST EXPECT IT

As soon as the shock wore off from the doctor's pronouncement, Mike and I gathered our things, put on our coats and exited the clinic. I had settled into an emotionless, hollow place. Yes, I had a game plan developing, but everything was still so new, so raw. Apparently, Satan was not finished with me just yet.

As we crossed the parking lot, a gust of wind pressed icy air against my cheeks as though it would penetrate right into my bones. I pulled my collar close. Unexpectedly I felt dark again and my legs started to shake. I stumbled and Mike tightened his grip on me. He stopped, looking over to see if I were all right. Seeing the change in my demeanor, he moved his hands to my shoulders and turned my body to face him. As I lifted my chin, our eyes met.

My body began convulsing uncontrollably and my voice dashed the silence. Mike pulled me closer as I heaved, and then my knees began to buckle. The shock from the reality of what we had just learned was settling into my consciousness.

Mike held me firm in his arms so that I would not fall and stated again in a somewhat unfamiliar voice, "It's going to be all right," and then he started to sob, too.

Both of us had held our emotions so close for so long. Not just for that day, but for the weeks and months previous. Questions and worry had invaded our minds creating a weight that was difficult, at best, to carry.

Grief wrapped its icy clutch around both of us. Mike buried his face into my hair and I thrust my mouth into the lapel of his coat trying to contain the sounds. Both of us trembled as our bodies expelled the trauma like a demon being exorcized. The darkness ebbed and flowed, in and out, right along with the windy vortex. It escalated and then suddenly tapered off. I let my imagination believe the ache was being whisked away with the blustery current.

As the breeze calmed, so did we. Mike leaned back, reached up with one hand and wiped his eye and asked, "Are you all right?"

I nodded and said, "I will be," not really sure if I would, but hoping it were the truth.

The grey clouds were still above us and perfectly imitated our current demeanor.

As I leaned against Mike, a glint of light caught my attention and I turned my head. A sliver of the orange sunset had carved its way through the bleakness and swathed us in warmth. I sighed heavily as it filled every crack that had just been created. It pacified me and I could breathe again. It was no coincidence that it came at that very second. *God sent it.* I was sure of it, and we needed it. I was reminded that He would never leave me completely alone, nor would He leave me comfortless. Gratitude soaked through me with the rays of the gilded light.

I lifted my eyes and noticed that Mike was also gazing west. The sun sparkled in his eyes and the look on his face told me he felt peace, too. I even thought I saw him smile a little.

He looked down at me, his eyes focusing intently. "I'm here … forever. You know that, right?"

A whoosh of air that sounded like a half cough expelled from my lips, and a tear fell, staining my cheek. All I could do was nod. Mike knew me so well. He knew exactly what I needed to hear, exactly when I needed to hear it. It had always been a gift he had, reading me like that. Another quality that I prized in him.

We stood still in the middle of that parking lot staring west, and with the last few remaining minutes of sunlight, we just held each other watching it fade.

My composure recovered, I pulled back and looked into Mike's eyes. "I love you," I said. "You know you're my rock? I couldn't have done this alone. Thank you for being here."

"Of course," he replied. "I love you! There was no way I was going to miss it."

He slipped his hand around my waist, turned and guided me toward the car. I glanced at my watch and realized I had a business meeting in an hour. I sighed, as hesitation flooded me.

"Are you going?" Mike said, knowing exactly what I was thinking.

I looked up at him tenuously, and instantly resolved to go. "The distraction will do me good," I muttered, not certain I would be able to keep my composure. Mike had to go back to work anyway; I hated the swing shift. It made more sense to spend the evening with familiar faces, than to go home alone with just my thoughts.

As we reached the car, he opened the door for me, swinging it wide, and then looked at me firmly repeating his earlier words, "I love you."

I smiled as much as my face would allow. It felt good to smile. The pent up tension released, leaving me feeling better. "I love you, too."

"We'll get through this," he said, his eyes piercing mine. "I want you to know, I'll be right here; I'm not going anywhere."

I heaved again and grabbed my mouth, tears attempting an encore. He had said it again, exactly what I needed to hear. He had no way of knowing that he was answering my fears. Just a few days earlier, I had been wrestling with the question of whether or not he would stay if it turned out that I had cancer. It felt silly to me now, that I had worried about it.

Mike hugged me tight, kissed me on the neck and then helped me into the driver's seat. "Right here," he said pointing toward my heart, "I'll be right here, no matter what."

As I reached for my seatbelt I said, "I love you."

"I love you, Alicia ..." and then he smiled, "always."

He stepped back and closed the door. My eyes had not left his. I really did not want to leave his side yet, but his break from work would be over in another ten minutes. He reached up, touching his fingers to his lips and then opened his hand toward me, giving me a kiss to carry. I smiled, said another "I love you," pulled out of the parking lot, and began driving south.

~

The hour-long drive gave me time to think. There was so much to process; my emotions were in chaos. As I vacillated back and forth between the multiple options, medical and otherwise, the waters became muddy and unclear and, for whatever reason, I had difficulty completely ruling out Dr. Calder's advice. Then the questions began.

"Do you honestly think you are so much better than other people that you can defy the entire medical community? Are you even emotionally strong enough? And what in the world are you going to do to heal your body? Do you even know? Most people trust medical science completely, so what is your problem? Why can't you just trust what everyone else does?"

Then the opposing side chimed in, "You're a strong woman. You've been through plenty of hard times. If this is what you feel good about doing, then you should do it. The information is out there somewhere; you just have to find it. Listen to your gut. What is it telling you?"

That last question made me feel better. My gut was telling me to explore every natural alternative I could unearth. I had no idea where I would find the information I needed or where to even start. I did not know if natural therapies actually worked, or how I would find those keys that would redirect my body back into a healthy state. I felt a little dumb because I was basing my decision off of instinct. But it still felt right. One thing I knew for sure—I wanted to live, and the doctor's proposals did not seem like life to me; they seemed like death.

Chapter Six

INITIALIZING THE CIRCLE

When I thought about who would be at the meeting, I decided I would keep my newly acquired information quiet, with the exception of Danica. She was my trainer, my mentor, and, most of all, my friend. It was not quite clear how I would tell her, but the fact that we worked closely together put her on a need-to-know basis.

I pulled into a parking stall, and before I got out of the car I took a moment to collect my thoughts. Leaning my forehead onto the back of my hands that were holding the steering wheel in a death grip, I began to pray.

I felt broken, and right then I needed deliverance from the enormity of my situation.

"Father," I began, "this isn't going to be easy, especially not tonight. Everything is so fresh. Please give me the strength to hold it together. I don't want to crack. I don't want to feel pressured into sharing my condition because I couldn't keep my emotions together." I breathed, lifted my head a little and scanned the parking lot. "I don't want to cry. Please just help me to not cry. Amen."

I stared out the front windshield when a tangible feeling started warming me from the inside out. It grew quickly until my skin tingled and the tension I had felt earlier, softened.

I closed my eyes again, "I really don't want to do anything the doctor recommended. It scares me. It just doesn't feel right," I muttered, turning my senses inward as I connected with the divine insights.

As quickly as I said it the thought came, "Then follow your heart."

It startled me. In fact, it confused me and I questioned it. "Really, but what if I die?" And as soon as I had said those words, they sounded silly. I was arguing with God. "Sorry," I said, "I heard you. If I follow my heart, then I'm going to do this naturally."

Opening my eyes, I looked across the steering wheel. "Well, if I don't follow my own heart, I'm sure other people will be happy to tell me what to do." I said, "I can do this." A surge of my positive mindset training kicked in. "I *can* do this!" I said a second time.

I was overwhelmed by the sensation that Jesus Christ was pleased with my decision. Peacefulness enveloped the air surrounding me and suddenly I knew He would support me.

I freshened my makeup and reached for the door handle, repeating my affirmation, "You can do this." At that I stepped out and crossed the parking lot with a surprising confidence.

I pulled the door open. The building was alive with activity. People were bustling about and lively chatting. Just ahead of me I saw Danica, who was happily visiting with a few other people. I called to her. She turned and smiled.

Danica stood about five-foot-two, but with her ever-shifting heel collection, she typically stood several inches taller than that. Her light-colored crystal green eyes sparkled, and she smiled wide, accentuating the dimples in her cheeks. I had always liked her, mostly because she had one of the most non-judgmental personalities I had ever encountered. She saw the good in most everyone and always had a positive word. I grew a little anxious as I approached, knowing what I was about to tell her would come as a shock.

When I reached her, I asked if I could talk to her privately. She nodded and quickened her step to follow me into a side hallway just out of view of the others who were gathering.

I turned to face her. Nervously I began to sweat and my heart palpitated, and for a moment the gloom from earlier seeped in. I wondered how in the world I was going to tell her.

I shifted my weight from one foot to the other, and lifted the notebook I had carried in, placing it in the crook of my arm. My heart was pounding. I was stalling and I knew it. Suddenly I lifted my eyes, connecting them with hers, and blurted, "I went to the doctor today."

I felt a bit like a scared animal. I searched for some sort of recognition in her eyes to my previous statement. I found it, her demeanor had changed and there was a shadow darkening the hue of her eyes. It sent an imaginary spear through my heart.

She squinted at me and said, "Oh?" The smile had faded from her face.

I wanted to reach out and hug her, and apologize, and somehow soften the blow of the news I was about to deliver. Instead I just stared at her.

Then all at once I was speaking. The delivery was so quick that I almost missed it. Carelessly, I heard myself announce, "I have breast cancer." It sounded sharp and insensitive. "Oh … that came out loud," I said, my voice cracking a little.

The words pierced me like someone had just plunged an ice pick into my throat. I already hated the exercise of telling people, and she was only the first. Her eyes dilated to three times their normal size and her mouth dropped open. Hastily she shut it and froze, staring at me.

It was not difficult to read her; she was stunned. I would have been in shock too if the tables had been turned. I scolded myself for being so callous.

"Geez, could you have said that any more pointedly? That was about as cold as it could have gotten. Dang it, Alicia! You should have said that more gently."

Half expecting Danica to burst into tears, I was surprised and thankful that her reaction was just the opposite. She actually smiled. It was a concerned, narrow smile, but a smile nevertheless.

"When did you find out?" she asked, trying not to sound stunned.

"About an hour ago," I responded in a strange, cool tone that made me seem like I was either in complete shock myself, or at peace with the entire thing.

She looked at me curiously, and said, "Why are you here?"

I looked at my feet again. I had already asked myself that question a hundred times. I forced a smile. Immediately I felt lighter, but the look on Danica's face was incredulous, and I expect my grin took her by as much surprise as it did me. She stared in disbelief.

Opening my mouth I began to explain, "Mike is working until nine so I decided it would be a good night *not* to be alone," And then, curiously, I laughed.

Danica looked shocked at my thought and then seemed to absorb my answer. I watched as the lines on her face softened. Her eyes narrowed and she asked, "What are you going to do?"

"I think I'm going to take the natural route," I said softly as a haze of confusion tiptoed into my brain.

Then just as quickly as that, she smiled a full, broad smile and exclaimed, "Wow. That's amazing. You're amazing!" My iffy confidence shifted with her declaration, and then she leaned in looking more serious and asked, "If I can help you at all, you'll let me know, right?"

"Of course," I said, "You'll be one of the first to know."

"Are you sharing the news with anyone else tonight?" she asked.

"No. Let's just keep it between us for now," I responded.

She nodded an affirmation, and I sighed, smiling from relief. I took note that my heart rate had returned to normal. Danica had not let me down. She was completely unaware that she was key to my future healing. She thanked me for telling her, hooked my arm with hers and then walked me toward the meeting room. Her hold was a bit cozier than I might have predicted, but it connected us. Love trickled out of her and right into me. It felt good to have an ally.

Chapter Seven

LIVING AS IF

Exhaustion. There was no other word for it. Both Mike and I looked a little like something the cat had dragged in: dark circles shading the skin beneath our eyes and very little spark left. I looked at the clock when I stepped into the kitchen, it was ten p.m. Mike had arrived only minutes before.

"I'm spent," I said, trying to rally enough energy to hug him and then climb the stairs to our bedroom.

Mike sighed heavily. "Me too," he said leaning into me, "You doing okay?"

I shrugged and lifted my arms to his neck and said, "As well as I could be. I told Danica."

"How'd that go?" he asked, leaning on me harder than I had strength for.

I mustered a bit more energy and pushed into him to regain my balance, "Really well, actually. She is going to be a good support." I said.

"Great," he responded.

We separated and trudged up the stairs. There was no more discussion about the situation that night. We readied for bed, and then knelt in prayer. Mike said it. It struck me that Mike's voice was deep and filled with pleading. As his words entered my ears, they settled on me in a layer of sadness, and that is how I slept, sullen and unsettled.

~

When I awoke in the morning, I could hear the shower running. Mike was awake. As I lay there, my chest felt as though someone had placed lead weights there.

I got up, put on my robe and went downstairs to the kitchen. Fifteen minutes later, Mike came into the room. He smiled at me, and then drew me into a stronghold. Gently he spoke in my ear, his breath heating my neck, "It's going to be all right."

I sighed. That was what I needed to hear. He had easily read my facial expressions and fed me the needed confidence. He had said it multiple times already, but just like a child, he would have to repeat it many times before the information could be fully absorbed. I definitely needed the repetition. I hoped he would say it a thousand times more. I lingered in his arms as long as I could. It was not long enough.

Far too soon, he pulled back, grabbed his lunch from off of the kitchen counter and headed toward the front door. I was close on his heels. "Everything is going to work out," he began. "Really. It's going to be fine." Then he smiled again and turned to leave.

"Love you," I said as I leaned on the door frame.

"Love you more!" he said, turning over his shoulder to look at me. I smiled and waved, and then he was gone.

Closing the door, I began to contemplate my day. I probably should have chosen to go shopping or something, for the distraction, but I did not. Instead, I got dressed and began cleaning. In fact, most of the day was spent in idle tasks that kept me from focusing too deeply. I felt quite lost. Even though I knew I had chosen to follow my heart, I still did not know how to accomplish the huge task at hand. I really did not have the first clue as to what steps I should take. My faith and trust in the Lord was growing, but I was still shaky. I knew Him well enough to know He would direct me in the right course, but was I strong enough to follow the promptings? I wondered.

Mike and I texted on and off during the day; he was sending words of encouragement as I was trying to keep my wits about me. It was a pretty difficult undertaking.

Things changed. My life was no longer easy and comfortable. Everything I had ever stood for was suddenly open for scrutiny, observation, and question. I examined myself. Did I really believe in Christ and did I truly think a simple phrase—*follow your heart*—was a heavenly sign? Was I willing to bet my life on it? It pressed against every shred of faith I had.

As I questioned myself, I quickly realized that every impulsive thought I had led me back to my foundation where prayer and trust in God were rudimentary. So I clung to that and decided to ask Mike for a blessing.

For most of my life, I had been in the habit of asking for blessings when things seemed too much for me to handle alone. In the past they had always given me solace and comfort. This truly was the test of all tests for me, though, and I knew it. I was familiar enough with the practice to understand that the counsel I might be given might not be what I wanted to hear. Would I listen and follow the divine, or would I falter and forge my own human path?

I picked my cell phone up from off the counter and sent a text to Mike. "I would like a blessing tonight," it read.

Moments later my phone vibrated and flashed the message, "You got it!" At the end of his remark he sent a smiley face, boosting my morale. Who would have thought that something as simple as a smiling yellow dot could lift my spirits?

As the day wore on, I thought about what might be said in the blessing and the courage it would take to accept the information with faith. In some ways it scared me to consider it. My degree of trust in the Lord was about to be revealed. What if I did not like what I heard? What if He instructed me to listen to my doctor's advice? Random musings wreaked havoc with me for the rest of the afternoon.

~

It was Saturday evening, a little over twenty-four hours since we had learned the news of my cancer. Mike arrived home around seven. He had called our neighbor, Steve, earlier in the day, asking if he would mind coming over to help give the blessing. At about eight o'clock, Steve knocked on the door.

I looked directly at Mike, my eyes instantly locked in fear about the idea of telling another person. Although I was closer to the door, I was unable to bring myself to rise from my chair and open it. I felt very tender and vulnerable and wondered what Steve's reaction would be.

As he stood there filling the door frame, Steve smiled pleasantly. He had always seemed humble, yet authoritative, and both Mike and I admired his spiritual strength. Each time he spoke there was kindness in his remarks. I believe he had a personal policy to leave people better than he found them because we always felt improved by his presence.

He stepped into the room. His gentle blue eyes gave me courage. I was still anxious about having to articulate my situation again but, strangely, I grew unexpectedly peaceful. He shook Mike's hand, and then mine, and after some idle chit chat he asked, "Do you mind if I ask what the blessing is for?"

I froze; the beating of my heart began to seriously outpace the rise and fall of my chest. I said nothing. I looked toward Mike who was choosing his words. The temperature in the room seemed to elevate, and my feet began to sweat. Mike knew that my silence was his signal to take over the conversation. He glanced at me and then back to Steve. With quiet emotion he stated, "Alicia has been diagnosed with breast cancer." I saw his jaw tighten slightly, which sent a twinge of pain through me.

My eyes darted to Steve. I studied his face. My tears were threatening to erupt. I felt awkward and on the spot. I anticipated a reaction of some sort from Steve, a gasp, a wince . . . something . . . but it did not happen. In fact, he did not even flinch. There was no noticeable response at all on his face. He continued

35

smiling and looked surprisingly undisturbed, as if he knew a secret I was not aware of.

He shifted his glance my direction and looked at me straight on with an intensity that disrupted the escalating distress I was feeling, instantaneously filling me with joy and love.

He said, "This is an opportunity for you to lean on the Lord harder than you ever have. Let the Atonement carry the burden."

He was so matter-of-fact that everything lifted like a fog after a rainstorm, and things grew clear. "Yes," I thought to myself, "this is a chance."

I immediately knew what to do. I had leaned on the Lord my whole life. I had leaned on Him harder the previous nine months while I wondered what the lump was. But now, I was filled with the distinct impression that it was time to rely on Him, absolutely, without wavering.

Confidence poured into me, and I was calm, ready and primed to hear whatever would be said in the blessing, knowing I would accept whatever the Lord's will was for me. Mike was the conduit. He, along with Steve, placed his hands on my head and said, "You will overcome this thing that has invaded your body, through your faith and diligence."

I held my breath. "I'm going to live?" Again, I shouted soundlessly, "I'm going to live!" and the tears began to spill down my cheeks. I could feel my body convulse and quickly attempted to hold it under control.

"Listen to those who love you and care for you, that this can be eradicated from your body," he continued.

Mike's voice resounded and permeated me, comfortingly, like a small child cuddled warm within a quilt. Again I replayed the word, "eradicated." It lingered there, evolving into solidly formed knowledge about my future. I felt warm and calm.

He continued, "Live as if it were not there."

Immediately I pictured future images: Christmases with family and friends where there was laughter and love, and presents tied with blue ribbons. I was so elated by the experience that I nearly forgot to listen to the rest of the blessing.

"Small procedure" came from Mike's lips, and then, "It will not return," tagged on the end. Hesitantly, I stepped away from the happy images to see if I had heard what I thought I had heard.

"Wait," I thought, willing myself to a halt. "What did you just say? In order to have it gone, I have to submit to a 'small procedure.' Is that what you said?"

My heart lurched and the joyful pictures faded in the background and went slightly out of focus, having lost position to this newly discovered image of a *procedure* I was forced to look at. I almost heard myself say, "No!" and then something odd happened.

There it was—my faith—open, exposed and wanting.

My open mind slammed shut and I tucked that phrase somewhere deep, pretending it had not been said.

Immediately I turned my attention on to positive things, even though I knew full well what had been said. I avoided looking at the "procedure" again for a long, long time … just like it was the plague. I had become efficient at personal mind control.

The blessing ended and Steve left. As Mike closed the door he turned and then took me into his arms. The pressure we had both felt, released. Then he said, his voice shaking, "I don't think the Lord is going to let you go. You have to stay here with me."

Mike held me there for the longest time, speaking softly in my ear; the heat from his breath distilling into my soul and mind.

And then I heard him mention the *procedure*. I snapped into reality like an elastic band, quick and sharp. Energy pulsed through my center and I emotionally stepped back changing the subject before Mike even realized I had done it.

I said, "How do you live 'as if' under these circumstances?"

Mike, who was entirely unaware of my deflection, said, "Just move forward with life and avoid spending too much time thinking negatively. But if you do have a hard day just sing. It always makes you feel better."

Sing. The word hit me like a full facial slap and I flinched. Aside from God and my family, it was the most important thing in my life. Instantly, I felt threatened because twice in my life I had lost my ability to sing. The memories flooded, troubling my spirit and reawakening the pain that had long since been suppressed. I squeezed my eyes shut, burying my face into Mike's shoulder, reliving them with eerie exactness.

The first was when I was twenty-one years old. I had been married for two years and was pregnant. Life seemed perfect with the anticipation of a baby, and then the unthinkable happened. I became horribly ill, coughing up blood in violent convulsions that shook me right down to my frame for several weeks. On a snowy Christmas morning, I went into premature labor and lost twin boys. I was twenty-four weeks along. The babies were born whole and beautiful and perfectly formed, but too early to survive. At the time, I thought I would most assuredly die from the grief, and the sting of their deaths haunted me for years. The physical symptoms, coupled with the emotional disturbance, created a situation where I lost my ability to sing for over two years. Life was hollow, and joyless.

On the other occasion, years after the first, I was helping a friend move out of her house. In a dark, unventilated cold storage room I was exposed to toxic fumes created by a cat litter box, which chemically burned my vocal chords, leaving me unable to sing for another two years.

"What if I lose the ability to sing again? Every time something really difficult has happened in my life, I've lost it," I whined in a sound that came out more high-pitched and fearful than I wanted it to. It blistered my ears with faithless inferences.

Mike pressed his cheek into my hair, reassuring me and saying, "It's going to work out. Your voice will be fine. You just need to keep singing every day, no matter what."

He always knew what to say. It was such a simple comment, but it was perfectly deposited, reconciling my fears. A quiet sigh slipped from my lips. He was right. If I just committed to sing everyday a couple of things would likely happen; my voice would have no choice but to stay in shape and my emotions would have a better chance of staying in check.

"Thank you," I whispered as the tension drained from my body and I allowed his body to meld into mine, satiating me with his love.

As the days passed and the shock of learning I had cancer wore down, I gained a little more restraint over my emotions. Life began to normalize in a peculiar way. Even though I managed to feel happy, I still struggled with the ugly ideas that would obviously plague me from time to time. Mostly it happened when the word *procedure* would find its way to the forefront, but I did not let it stay. I pushed it out each and every time, and because I did not *feel* sick, it was easy to get on with living my life and to forget about everything.

Chapter Eight

BREAKING THE NEWS

I am embarrassed to admit that it took me days to call my parents. Somehow, it was the most difficult tasks to consider. Mom had gone through something very similar fifteen years earlier. Honestly, it was not her feelings I was considering, it was my own selfishness. I did not want to hear about her experience with radiation.

I was acutely aware that my parents knew nothing about the blessing I had received. I was also aware of their love and care for me, so if I were to open that door too far, they might influence me into a course of action I was opposed to. I had always trusted them, and the possibility of their recommendations diverting my chosen direction terrified me.

One day I drove around aimlessly for a long time before calling them, contemplating what I would say. After avoiding it as long as I could, I parked in the most peaceful out-of-the-way spot I could find. The last unforgiving gust of winter was hanging on and pretty much mirrored how I was feeling that afternoon: icy, exposed and stark.

I folded my forearms on the upper most part of the steering wheel and leaned onto them, uttering a little prayer. After I composed what I wanted to say, I dialed the phone. My body was shaking and I suddenly felt cold even though the car heater was blowing at full capacity.

It rang twice and Mom answered cheerfully. I could hear the engine of their car.

I tried to match her tone by sounding as cheery as I could and asked, "Hey, could you guys pull over somewhere? I have something really important I want to talk to you about." I prayed that my voice would hold steady and not give away my escalating trepidation.

As soon as she indicated that they had stopped, I said, "I'm going to tell you something very important and I don't want you to say anything until I'm completely finished." My heart started pounding harder.

"Okay. Oh, hang on just a sec ... okay. It's on speaker," she said cheerfully as if she thought what I was going to say was something happy or fun, or playful.

I feel bad now for what my words may have sounded like on their end of the phone. I pretty much bulldozed my way through the one-sided conversation, talking so fast that there was no room left for questions or comments from them.

"Um, uh," I stammered as my blood pressure began raging. "I have something to say, and I don't want you or Dad to talk until I'm completely finished." I pressed on, "I went to the doctor the other day; I have breast cancer."

I did it again! Throwing that phrase around like I was asking for a second helping of pie! It shocked me how coarse it sounded every time I verbalized it. I was beside myself with fury and irritation that the words were attached to me. I felt sick.

I heard a gasp and pictured Mom grabbing her mouth to stop any other noises from expelling themselves. She had always gone out of her way to avoid anything that would hurt me, and here I was just blowing a hole through her chest without so much as a "how do you do."

I knew full well my parents would take extraordinary measures to adhere to my request of not speaking as I had asked. I knew they would avoid saying anything unless I asked directly, simply *because* I asked; in fact, I was banking on it. Their adherence was all that was holding me together. Any word from them and I think I would have crumbled.

Rather than allowing them time to process what I had just said, I pressed on with an urgency that probably left them feeling rather frenzied, because that is exactly what I felt.

With powerful and firm resolve I said, "I don't want you guys to ask me about it." I choked on my own words and caught myself in a heave that threatened to overcome the delicate balance I had formed. "I don't want you to give me any suggestions or thoughts as to what I should or shouldn't do. I need positive energy from you and prayers *only*."

The voice I heard was rough, and did not sound like mine. I wanted to throw both my arms across my mouth and stop. I wanted to listen to my mother's voice kindly telling me that everything would be okay. I wanted to let them both comfort and soothe me. But I could not, not yet. There was no stopping now. I had to press on, and I did it with such abandon that it felt like it was burning a hole right through the skin of my belly. I needed to vomit.

If for some reason Mom or Dad had interjected at this point and asked me to consider the medical option, I might have done it. In truth, I did not want anyone attempting to sway me into whatever decisions I was going to make. I knew that my parents had the power to convince me of anything, but I simply did not give them the chance to offer any advice. Although I had already made up my mind, I still felt tenuous and somewhat weak about it. My parents would support whatever I chose, but I was not about to allow them a chance to try so I kept talking.

"If I bring it up or *ask* for your advice, feel free to give it to me—but not unless I ask."

And that was it. Every word came out in a rush, like a fire hose violently discharging to put out a fire. But that is not what was happening. The flames were not being extinguished; I was throwing gasoline onto them. I had ignited my parents' imaginations to a reality they were already familiar with. Not only was I dumping this unthinkable weight on them, there was now a chasm between us that shut down any and all communication, and I was the master of its creation.

As the words were rolling off my tongue, I realized just how deeply I had stepped into self-preservation mode. I quailed at the force at which I had so systematically excluded my parents from open discussion about my situation. I was wrapping my emotions tight like a cocoon, and if or when I was ready, I would emerge, but not before. I guess it was the only way to produce a modicum of mastery over what felt was an out-of-control state of affairs.

I continued talking for a long time, telling them how I planned on holistically treating myself, the things I had heard in my blessing, what the doctor had said, how I felt about it all. I tried to sound in command, hoping it would not betray the fact that I was on the verge of tears. I'm positive they read right though it all, but they said nothing, and simply listened.

After my ten-minute tirade was over, I stopped talking and waited for a response. I could hear Dad sighing heavily in the background, a sound I knew all too well whenever he was upset about something. My heart ached and my whole body trembled.

All there was on the other end of the phone was silence. Pain was the next thing I felt; it was my mother's. I could hear her halting breath. It was almost a gasp, like she was ordering her tears to stay put. When she finally breathed in as though she had something to say, I heard her stop again, hesitating. Then she drew in another breath and spoke, simply saying "Okay. We love you." I could hear the same shake in her voice that I was hiding.

"I love you guys, too," I said, wondering if they could believe that I did after just decimating them both. "Thanks for listening. I'll touch base with you later," I said, shutting the call down before everything I was holding in erupted.

Hanging up, I dropped my phone on the passenger seat and grabbed the steering wheel again, this time I curled my hands around it like I was pulling it into a hug. I hit my forehead against the rim two or three times, shrieked, and then bawled for a long time, until my sides hurt.

I do not remember how I even got home later. All I know is that I found myself on the couch, curled into a ball, and buried under a blanket.

Chapter Nine

THOSE WHO LOVE AND CARE FOR YOU

Even though I had decided not to accept any traditional therapies when I had consented to the MRI, there was that tiny splinter of possibility remaining that I might consider *some* of the doctor's recommendations. So at the time they offered it, I felt like I had to explore that last piece of evidence, just to be sure.

I could feel the hostility rise within me again as I was shown to the doctor's office to receive the results. In truth, I did not want to talk to or see her again. She represented something dark and deadly.

I bowed my head in the silence of the doctor's office and began to pray, knowing that God was the only one who could deliver me from the sensations brimming inside. Suddenly, there was a knock and the door rattled open. Dr. Calder burst in, stealing away any offering heaven might have given. My eyes shot up and met hers.

She greeted me with that same lifeless, empty "Hello." To me she resembled a robotic drone, moving through the room as though it were some kind of prison sentence.

Within about three minutes I realized she was not having a conversation with me; she was peddling her wares! She discouraged the less expensive and less invasive *procedure;* the lumpectomy, and sped right over to the most expensive and impactful item on her list—a double mastectomy.

She said, "The lump is the size of a key lime. If we were to remove it, you would not be happy with the cosmetic result."

I asked the obvious question, "Don't they have implants to fix something like that?"

"No," she said emphatically without further explanation. "I would advise you to have a double mastectomy," she said callously, without any thought to what she was suggesting.

It hit me with great force, as if the very powers of heaven were streaming the thought directly into my mind, "She just said that a double mastectomy would be a better cosmetic outcome than a lumpectomy." I should have laughed, but I bit my tongue.

Almost without thought I felt my body harden as I grew angrier by her insensitivity. By looking at me she would not have noticed unless she were an expert at reading the darkening shades of green that I could feel intensifying in my eyes. She spoke with such ease, with absolutely no emotion attached, no compassion, just frosty, hard facts. I *tried* to remember any previous kindness and to understand how hard her job might be. But I decided that *her* plight did not faze me in the least; I did not care what she had to do every day. She had chosen her profession, and I was free to choose my life.

Dr. Calder continued talking incessantly while I mentally disengaged from the torrent of data being heaped upon me, and began thinking about how dark she looked. Her skin was sallow and the circles under her eyes matched the dull grey in her hair. She leaned forward, toward me, trying to engage. It was probably due to the fact that I had glassed over and was not really listening to her. I tried to appear as though I had reengaged, but in truth I remained intentionally distant.

Calculating my next question, I asked, "What would you do if you were me?" My voice sounded cool.

"I'd have a double mastectomy," she said, sliding back into her chair, flinching ever so slightly, and then locking eyes with me again.

"She's lying," I said, starting an internal conversation with myself. "Dr. Calder does *not* love or care for me."

The words boomed, and the darkness that had pervaded earlier immediately and completely fell away with a rush of confidence that suffused me. It took all I had to not stand up and walk out the door that very moment. I sat up straight, governing the speed of my movements, thanked her for her time, and told her I would consider her proposals. Then I stood, walked to the door and left.

Maybe it was limited thinking on my part to walk away from standard treatments; after all, 98% of the general population believe it to be the *only* thing to do. But I was following my heart and it said to leave, slam the door shut, and run for my life. . . literally.

As I pushed the glass doors open and stepped into the sunlit, snow-covered parking lot, I resolved to stick with the advice of those who loved and cared for me. I knew God loved and cared for me. Mike loved and cared for me. Mom and Dad loved and cared for me. Danica loved and cared for me. I would listen to them.

I silently said a prayer of gratitude. It did not go unnoticed that God was the One who nudged me out of that situation with Dr. Calder.

Dr. Calder's office called me nearly every day for two weeks. I ignored every call, letting them go to voicemail. Every message sounded more serious and urgent than the previous.

I was stubborn, and glad of it. Every day things became a little less hazy. I was moving away from fear and more firmly into faith, becoming more actively involved in finding my own solutions, which gave me a huge sense of control. That, in turn, shaped a solid firmness regarding my plan to heal naturally. It would be another ten months before I saw another doctor. The rebel in me was alive and well. I felt a little smug about that.

Chapter Ten

GATHER GATHER GATHER

Over the next few weeks I told others in my circle who loved and cared for me about my situation. There were only ten initially. As I discussed my desire to do things naturally, every last one of them agreed to my logic and encouraged me, giving me greater confidence.

On three separate occasions, however, I chose to come out of my shell and tell someone outside that intimate circle of confidants. Each would tell tales of people they knew who had suffered from cancer, what had happened and how it affected them.

The owner of a small store told me about his neighbor who had breast cancer a few years previous. Not knowing what to do, I froze in silence. Mentally I searched for something else to focus on. Oddly, I landed on the Alphabet Song, silently singing it while smiling at him as if I were listening intently. It was my first experience with thoughtless, inconsiderate dialogue.

The second was a clerk in a health food store who was showing me the benefits of juicing. As she crushed an apple in the machine, she aimlessly told of a close friend who had "lost her battle with cancer" and how it had impacted their family, how devastated they all were, how it had broken her heart, how she cried about it for weeks. I thought she was going to shed a tear right there. Singing the Alphabet Song did not work that time. My jaw dropped slightly in astonishment, and I felt a little like an old, wrung out wash rag by the time she finished. It took me three hours of positive affirmations *and* a strawberry smoothie to get over that one!

Then there was Rob. I had only met him briefly in person a few times so I cannot call him a friend. He was more of a business mentor. We had been introduced by a mutual colleague and spoke briefly via cell phone each week regarding business. As soon as he heard my news, he began to detail the awful situation his niece found herself in. She had an aggressive form of cancer and was deeply involved in mainstream medical treatments. He described the large clumps of hair that were falling out of her head due to the chemotherapy she was undergoing.

He was the last person to knowingly share such information with me because I never allowed it again. As for Rob, I am afraid I lashed out rather harshly at him on the phone. In anger I rhetorically asked, "Rob ... why are you telling me this? What is wrong with you?" It sort of shocked me and sent a rush of voltage coursing through my veins. I raised my voice to a level that had rarely escaped me before. Loud and forcefully I continued, "I don't need to hear that kind of stuff right now! Do you realize how hard it is to listen to stories like this in my current circumstance? Do you have any clue what you're even doing right now? I don't want to hear anymore. Please stop!"

If embarrassment were measurable, I was in the red zone. Certainly my outburst would have caused Rob to feel very embarrassed, but mine was registering at a full-on ten. I forced my lips together and squeezed them tight just in case I was tempted to have another outburst. I sat in utter shock at my uncharacteristic behavior.

I heard a distinct gulp on the other end of the line. Rob was clearly startled by my eruption. He stuttered an apology. "Oh ... uh," and then he spurted, "I, I, am so, so sorry."

For a very uncomfortable few seconds no one spoke. I was angry, mostly at myself for telling him about the cancer in the first place. I was my own worst enemy. Why did I not just keep my mouth shut? Obviously it was too late to erase the images of Rob's nearly bald niece, but I had brought it on myself by opening the door. The pictures were now burned indelibly into my memory.

It was probably cruel of me to do it, but all I said was, "I appreciate your apology, Rob. Good-bye!" And at that I hung up the phone with a resolve to never speak to him again. My hands were shaking so badly that I dropped my phone.

It was then I vowed to avoid any and all conversations with anyone outside of my small and cherished circle. That proved to be one of the best and most valuable strategies that I implemented.

Another powerful lesson I gleaned was that dark forces could and would use anyone to castigate me—at any time—whether I told them about my situation or not. More times than I can count, random conversation would begin with people who came into my life; people I knew and many I did not. They somehow would find their way around to telling cancer stories without knowing the particulars of my life at all. It was just ordinary conversation to them. I could be in a group talking about shoes, and suddenly the conversation would shift to cancer. I speedily learned how to tune those stories out completely by counting to ten or singing silently. I learned to recognize the source, which helped me see reality a little more clearly. There was only one being who wanted me weak and scared. Yes, Satan is clever.

Something else happened as well. Awareness began to fill me as I realized how far-reaching cancer had become. I had done very little study on cancer and its impact on the general population so one afternoon I opened my laptop and typed in "cancer statistics." It rocked me to the core to realize that one in three people would be diagnosed with cancer during their lifetime[1] and the numbers were steadily increasing.

---

[1] http://goo.g1/7I9iKR for information regarding current cancer death rates.

That piqued my interest and my studies began. On a daily basis I would search the Internet and things began to line up. I began to realize how much I had to learn. It was daunting as there were massive amounts of information; however, I was pretty motivated.

One of the best pieces of advice I received was from one of my confidants. He said, "Just gather, Alicia. Gather, gather, gather! Gather all the information you can . . . all of it—the good and the bad." And that is exactly what I ended up doing.

For days I read and researched, and then finally after quite a bit of time I realized that the *only* way I could ever actually heal was to create the internal environment to heal by boosting my immune system. However, I could *not* rely on man-made chemicals. They were not capable of healing; they were specifically designed to *kill* something.

What a profound shift in my thinking.

When I grasped this fully, I set to work digging through the personal blogs and websites of *real* people who had overcome cancer. I went on Internet sites where holistic ideas were embraced. I was in full gathering mode and nothing was going to stop me.

It surprised me how diametrically opposed each side of the cancer argument was. One side was saying stay away from medical treatment, while the other was telling me to embrace it. It was indicative of how I felt most days—like a rollercoaster. "No wonder people get so confused," I told myself. Clearly, I was not interested in the medical information and was quite leery of it, but it did give another perspective, which did nothing but harden my courage and resolve to heal without it.

As my confidence grew, I let go of the day to day whiney "why me" prayers and instead I fell into the habit of asking, "What next?"

It became a little uncanny, really. People that I met would say something, igniting an inspired thought. Or, one of my friends would introduce me to someone who had the knowledge I needed. Answers to my natural-treatment questions were handed to me nearly every day, most times without the deliverer even realizing it.

Chapter Eleven

TITANIUM IS NOT ORGANIC

Several weeks had passed since I had learned about my breast cancer, and I noticed that the tumor began to change. Fear lurched within my heart and then the pounding began.

"Oh no." The words infiltrated. "Is it bigger?"

"Did I miss something? Maybe I'm on the wrong track!" A sick, empty feeling escalated within me, overtaking any logical thinking. The feelings and this logic clashed in a battle of irrational, nonsensical reasoning.

"Maybe there is nothing I can really do. Maybe it's all subjective to life and my efforts are in vain. Maybe God is displeased with my choices." I felt faint. The sick feeling began to make its way into my throat. I heaved, stopping short of vomiting.

"Are you okay?" Mike asked from the other room, looking concerned.

I grabbed the cup from off the counter and filled it with water then drank.

"I don't know," I said in a tenuous tone. "I need a second opinion."

"With what?" he asked, trying to catch up with my line of thought.

"I need you to check the tumor," I said, trying not to sound alarmed.

He noticed. "What's wrong?" he quizzed.

I looked at him. His brow had creased and his eyes had grown a deep shade of cobalt.

"Just check it," I said, not answering his query. I watched the shade of his skin shift from light to dark as realization filled him. Then he spoke, "There's no question; it's bigger."

I cringed and my heart sank into a dark space. Suddenly I felt like throwing up again. Then questions engulfed me one more time, "Are all my efforts wasted? Is it too late to change the direction of my cancer? Maybe Dr. Calder was right; maybe I should have listened to her."

The queasy feeling churned hot in the middle of my stomach and I wondered if I were to retch, would I even make it to the toilet? Tears seared the back sides of my eyes and then began falling freely. Fear swelled in me like a wave coming in with a tsunami. I felt defeated.

I reached for Mike, pulling him as close as I could get. His warmth quieted me, and then just as subtle as could be, the words from the blessing I had received came to me, "Live as if."

Fighting the urge to slide backward where I might moan and cry, I squeezed my eyes shut and gave my anxiety a shove. "You will *not* derail me today!" I said silently, bristling against the emerging feelings. "I'm going to live *as if* and I'm going to heal!"

A huge sigh hissed between my teeth until I was completely empty of air, and then I pulled away from Mike and sat on the edge of our bed. The space between us was still. I felt my eyes glaze over, and then Mike touched my forearm as he sat down next to me.

"I'm supposed to *live as if*," I said.

I looked over at him. He smiled kindly and said, "It's going to work out. I know it's going to work out. It may not seem that way now, but God never lies. I never got the feeling that you were going to die during that blessing. We have to have faith."

I nodded as he leaned into me. "Are you going to be all right?" he quizzed gently, knowing that he had to leave for work and hoping he would not have to leave me in need.

"I will be. You're right; it's going to be fine." The thumping in my chest subsided. It was like the Lord was telling me that my thinking was correct.

"I don't want to leave you unless you're sure you're going to be all right," he said.

"No, I'll be fine. I just needed to be reminded," I responded.

"I love you, you know that right?" Mike asked.

I smiled. That was one thing I did know. "Yes," I said. "And I am so grateful."

Standing, he pulled his keys from his pocket and said, "I'll text you later, but don't hesitate to text or call me if you need me. I'll have my phone close."

"Okay," I said as I stood to walk him to the door.

"And for heaven's sake, keep yourself busy and make sure you sing today," he instructed as he opened the front door.

"I love you," I said, trying to look cheerful.

"I love you, too. Everything is going to be fine," he said. Then he smiled and left.

He barely had time to get into the car when my phone beeped with a text from him saying, "Focus on living *as if.*" I smiled at his persistence regarding my mental state.

~

Countless times that day I prayed, not just inaudibly while performing whatever task I was involved in but literally down on my knees in humble, answer-seeking prayer. Even though I knew the words to my blessing, I still felt so vulnerable. I knew that God understood me and what I was dealing with so I did not hesitate to spend time talking with Him. I just felt like I needed more clarification. It completely baffled me that after nine months of no change in the tumor, it was now noticeably growing. Why?

A spark flickered causing me to run to my computer to check the impression. I began clicking through numerous blogs and medical sites about the practice of biopsies for diagnosis. The answers were there. Several sites confirmed what I was thinking. It sickened me.

Something entered my body via the needle from the biopsy, not only poking a hole in the protective outer casing of the tumor where affected cells could escape, but leaving something behind—the titanium clip. That clip, from the best of my ability to learn, had begun to wreak havoc on the tumor. In response, the tumor was beginning to morph.

For a while I stared blankly at the information, numbness setting in. A hum, like the sound of a chainsaw engine whirred in the distance somewhere. Facts, they were right there on the computer screen in front of me. My tear-blurred vision focused as the suggestions moved forward into perfect clarity for me to examine. I could barely process the information.

My first thought was of Caleb, who had positioned that tiny piece of metal in my breast in the first place. Anger scorched my skin and my eyes opened, draining a steady stream of tears that ran down like acid.

Then things shifted like sand under my feet and I remembered that it was still not Caleb's fault. As much as I wanted to blame him for this, it was not his doing—it was mine. I was the one who chose to have that test done. That was it. A sick nausea came over me.

I threw myself across the cushions of the couch and began wailing and sobbing in a manner that would have brought a grown man to his knees. Shrill sounds splintered the quiet of the room, shaking my whole body. Time passed, but I had no idea how much. Then, I stopped.

Drained, I pulled in a divided gasp, sat up and lumbered to the bedroom, decidedly trying to escape the pain that hung in my living room like thick smoke.

Reaching the bed, I doubled over near the edge, falling into a mass on the floor. Comprehending the effects of the clip being inserted into the tumor pounded until my realization was complete. I felt broken and buried. I began praying and openly begging, "Please, Father, help me! Please, please help me."

Pressing my forehead into the comforter that hung over the mattress, I steadied enough to hear a quiet word pass by my ears: "Forgive." Then it happened a second time, more forcefully than the first, and I distinctly heard the word, "Forgive."

It was not a surprise that I heard an actual word; spiritual experiences like this had happened in my life from time to time. The fact that they were rare was the reason it got my attention. I held my breath. It did not seem an easy task to forgive Caleb; it was his carelessness and neglect in articulating what he was doing that had brought me here.

Then realization slapped me one more time. It was not Caleb who needed forgiving; it was me.

Humbled and broken, I thought about what I was sensing. Deflecting my frustration to Caleb was a defense mechanism, a transfer of responsibility. In my weakness I had agreed to the tests so it was me who was to blame for the outcome I was now faced with.

A still, ever-so-small whisper fluttered near me a third time—"Forgive." I drew in a hiccup-sounding breath that nearly gagged me. I shook my head as I realized what I had to do. I prayed again, "Please. . . ." I faltered. "Please, please help me," I began again, and then said, "I forgive you, Alicia."

And then I began crying again. It was all I could do to absolve myself. As I allowed the feelings of forgiveness to enter my soul, I released. My body relaxed as if it were being thawed from a very long, very cold winter. Moments later I felt as if I were being washed by a summer rain and began to feel better, lighter. Ever so slowly I let go of the self-condemnation.

Then I understood; God was still there. I could feel Him. He had not gone away, nor had He lied to me in my blessing. He had not promised the road would be simple; He had promised that I would "overcome this thing." As my courage returned, I concluded that He was still going to fulfill his promise to me of healing; all I had to do was move forward and have faith.

That day I learned that Christ would step in whenever I needed Him. I grew to understand that He would help me move through each difficulty, and that He would be ever-patient with my slow learning curve. The desire to blame myself, or anyone else, fell away from my consciousness.

Chapter Twelve

THE BODY IS NOT A TRASH COMPACTOR

After God reaffirmed His will for me, I reacquired my courage and set out to change a few things. If I accepted as truth that He would heal me, I had to do my part. I took it upon myself to overhaul my diet by taking Mike's advice when he said, "It's your body, you can do whatever you want." I had to do everything in my power to change the nutritional imbalance in my body.

One afternoon I sat down and carefully inspected what I had been eating. As I wrote things out, I recognized changes that had to be made. I also realized that when the inorganic item from the biopsy was introduced into my body, bad things happened. It did not take a Master's Degree to figure out that I should be putting organic foods into my organic body.

I swore off of sweets, meat, and anything artificial or covered in pesticides. Fast food was kicked off my list, along with anything processed. Preservatives, GMOs, and anything that was altered from its original state were removed. I examined what was left—just the bare, down-to-earth basics, literally. What was left was that which came directly from the earth. Immediately I began a regime of eating fruits, vegetables, nuts, seeds and whole grains.

One afternoon while I was juicing a pile of apples and carrots, my phone rang. It was Marilyn, one of my carefully selected inner circle of friends. We had known each other for a few years, had traveled together and spent time just having fun. She was also Danica's mother. It made for a very favorable trio.

She said, "I have someone I would like to introduce you to. His name is Cowboy Don Tolman, the Whole Foods Medicine Man."[2]

I pressed my cell phone tighter to my ear and said, "What? You mean that's what his name is?"

Marilyn chuckled. "That's what they call him. Anyway, he's pretty well-known and he has a philosophy about food that is a lot like yours."

It surprised me a little that she thought I had a philosophy about food— I really had not clearly defined it for myself yet, but it made me smile that it was prominent enough to be noticed.

I wondered how anyone with a name like Cowboy Don, would have anything of interest for me. "Okay, sure," I said. "Tell me more."

"My daughter Chelsey worked for him a few years ago," Marilyn said as I heard a dish clang against the sink she must have been standing at. "She says he's an awesome guy and really smart. He's worked with a lot of people and Chelsey says they claim some pretty impressive healing stories. Some even claim he helped them learn how to cure their cancer."

She had my interest. "What? Seriously? How in the world did he do that?" I asked.

"I don't know, but he does consultations so there's really nothing to lose if you want to meet him. Are you game?" Marilyn quizzed.

I hesitated as my skepticism, not to mention my cynicism started a mini-war inside my brain. My brow creased and confusion clouded my judgment for a second. "There is a cure for cancer?" I caught myself asking silently. "How could there be a cure and no one's ever heard about it?" Then I caught myself—of course, there *had* to be! I completely believed that or I would have taken the doctor's advice and started chemotherapy immediately.

---

[2] For information on Don Tolman visit www.thedontolman.com (name and title used by permission).

Logic prevailed and I knew I had to be open to any and all *gathering*, so I agreed to the meeting, wondering if I would be the next victim of one of those "do-it-today-and-get-50%-off" pitches. The dialogue going on in my head confirmed my cynicism, "You just committed to listen to a self-proclaimed *whole food medicine man*, Alicia. Either you're crazy or he is."

For all of five seconds I listened to the internal argument and then simply agreed to the consultation. "Okay," I said to Marilyn. "Let's do it. I certainly have nothing to lose."

~

Two days later I met up with Marilyn at her place and we drove twenty minutes to Park City. She pulled into the parking lot of a small shopping center where we were meeting Don. It looked legitimate enough—a nice little storefront just off of the freeway. As I reached out and pulled the front door open, the nasty voices in my brain were slamming my decision to be there. As we entered the store, I told them to "shut up" and reminded myself to keep an open mind.

Inside it was open and airy, with large windows that let the sunlight in. It was clean and uncluttered, and our voices echoed. I looked around. Standing in the back corner near some small tables stood a cowboy, presumably Don. He was quite the picture. He was wearing a striking black cowboy hat, black jeans, a black and tan western shirt . . . and tennis shoes. That threw me off a little and I smirked; I expected boots. His closely shaved beard was silver on the sides and chin, and black where his mustache was, which extended right down to his jaw line.

"Wow," I thought to myself, "he *is* a cowboy."

My apprehension about him dissolved immediately as he shook both our hands as if we were long-lost friends. Then he walked us to a table that sat just out of the sunlight. As we sat I noticed a young man and woman quietly visiting on the opposite side of the warehouse-sized room.

After introductions, Marilyn and I detailed my health issues. I hated having to listen to it itemized so openly. I cringed inside, feeling the awkwardness of sharing something so personal with a perfect stranger. My skin grew cold and a nervous shake began vibrating right in the center of my stomach, causing me to lay my hand there for a moment.

Then Don looked at me, transfixing me with an aura of strength and his seemingly genuine concern. Then he spoke, "Yer gonna be all right, Little Missy." His confidence, along with his country drawl, drew me right in as though he were a concerned friend sharing something of importance with me. My queasiness was instantly calmed. He spoke of natural healing, eating foods from the earth, fasting, and lifelong health. He talked of lost knowledge from ancient times, about the restoration of bodily function, of eating fruits and vegetables in their season, and of whole foods and grains.

My ears tingled with the truth of his words. It was familiar information I had learned from studying scripture. He talked for forty-five minutes straight about the ancient ways of healing and how he literally traveled and searched the world for seventeen years for the answers he now possessed.

For all those years of studying and searching and *gathering*, one thing had eluded him; it was the meaning of a word he had heard in a Sunday School class when he was eight years old—the word was "Pulse." It came from the book of Daniel. He told me he had discovered what it was from a translated stack of writings that were packaged inside a wooden crate from a museum in London.

"What are the odds?" I wondered.

"Also in the box was the original papyrus scroll the translation came from, rolled up in a glass vial, sealed at the ends with wax," he detailed.

I became aware that my mouth was open and I was staring, a little in disbelief but mostly in fascination. His knowledge impressed me and the information he laid out for me was very convincing.

"It took me all that time to figure out what Pulse was!" He stated, "And I learned it was fruits and veggies, nuts and seeds. The things that are healthy for us to eat are so simple that people miss it."

Everything he said resonated with me. I do not think I disconnected from him the entire time we were there. It was like he was feeding me with the verification I needed to forge ahead holistically; yet I was still filled with apprehension.

My attention moved to the front door as it made a noise. An older couple walked through, disrupting our conversation. Don smiled at them and waved. They lingered near the door, and Don told us the two were his next appointment. As he wound the conversation down and thanked us for coming, he stood, preparing to end our discussion.

I instinctively grabbed the edge of the table, subconsciously demanding that he stay. I was so disappointed at the abrupt ending that I almost said something that likely would have come out wrong. I caught myself before the words escaped. All of a sudden I felt frantic and my eyes glassed over. My knuckles were turning white. I almost reached out and grabbed his wrist in a last-ditch effort to convince him to stay. Instead, I contained my emotions and shoved them into a cubby hole.

I released the table, followed Don's lead, and stood. I felt like someone had just handed me a silver platter, but took the dessert off before I got a hold of any. Surprisingly, just as I was getting my wits about me, Don leaned in and gave me a bear hug, and then stated, "I'm a hugger." He did the same with Marilyn while smiling broadly. As we walked toward the door, he put a hand on my shoulder. "Thank you so much for coming," he said in that southern-style drawl. Then added, "Yer awesome!"

Don stepped towards the older couple, arms outstretched, embracing each of them in turn and introducing them to us as Tom and Barbara.

"Tom here," Don said gently, patting him on the shoulder, "used to have prostate cancer."

To which Barbara said, "Yes, until we met Don." She was looking at Marilyn as she said it. "And now he doesn't have it anymore!"

Don laughed and then stepped away to where the younger couple I had noticed earlier was standing.

Barbara turned toward me and asked, "Are you here to get cured by Don?"

Choking on her boldness, I said nothing. Gratefully Marilyn chimed in, "Yup, we're here to get cured," she said with a chuckle.

Barbara then looked over her left shoulder toward Don and said in a loud voice, "Well, if you do what he says, you'll get better!" She then excitedly began telling us about her husband, who seemed perfectly happy to let her do the talking. He just stood there grinning from ear to ear. As she told their story, she went on and on about Tom's recent testing and how the doctors could not explain his recovery, when just a few months before they were announcing his impending death.

I was mesmerized and my jaw dropped slightly at her declarations. It hit me that this was the first time I had heard a story of natural healing directly from the source. I was awestruck. Electricity coursed through me and re-solidified my decision to restore my health naturally.

I looked past Barbara to focus on Don who was chatting and laughing with the young couple, and I was wonderstruck, internally questioning if he had really delivered enough information to help cure Tom. The strongest desire in me at that moment was to ask them all of the questions that were sprinting across the screen of my mind. My tongue was on the edge of conversation; however, I bit it, unwilling to tip my hand about my cancer to another stranger.

I was flooded with disappointment when the conversation with Barbara ended. I had most definitely not collected everything I wanted. Regretfully, we walked to the glass doors. I felt like I was pulling a fifty-pound sack of flour behind me. I lumbered forward and exited the building. I had just stepped away from something really important; I could feel it. I did not know if or when I would ever speak to Don again, but before I left Marilyn that day, I got Don's home- and cell-phone numbers with a resolution to find a way to be in his company again and to learn more about what he knew.

Later that very afternoon, I intentionally sent a message of gratitude to him, via text, for what he had taught me. It unlocked a sliver of communication between us. I yearned to have it develop into friendship over time, because I knew I could not afford his consultation fees, nor did insurance cover it—not that we had any anyway.

I did not know it then, but Don held one of the final keys to begin my healing process.

Chapter Thirteen

CONSPIRING MEN

Autumn hit in a dramatic explosion of red and gold tones that dripped from the trees like butter. I almost missed it due to the hours I spent staring at the computer screen reading. Along with the change in the season, a change in my perspective came as I began to grasp the incomprehensible reality that there were people out there who would exploit me and my situation for money.

As I read and studied, I gained a clear understanding of something I had never considered before; our food supply had become tainted to a rather large degree. It was no longer the food that God had created.

From genetically-modified to pesticide-covered, I learned that I had unwittingly been ingesting foods that were unhealthy for my system. Yes, I had changed my diet to be more in line with nature, but even then, nature had been tampered with.

I spent countless hours digging through websites, reading and cross-referencing scriptures that supported the ideas I had developed, and pored over books that held information that piqued my interest and supported my intended direction of action. My greatest gain, however, came from reading the words of Christ and His prophets.

No amount of outside information supported what I was doing for my health more than the scriptures. It buoyed my faith and lifted my thought processes to a point that assured me I was on the right road, even though I still struggled. Like Daniel, I was learning how to not defile my body with substances that could damage it.

One particular day a phrase came to me, almost like a whisper blowing past my ears—"conspiring men." It was a bit random, but I paid attention, knowing this was typically how spiritual revelation came to me. I had worked to hone my listening abilities since my initial diagnosis, learning that the Lord would guide me if I paid enough attention to the promptings he freely offered.

As the odd thought about conspiring men settled, I grabbed a rag that hung across the faucet, and aimlessly began wiping the kitchen counter, mentally trying to understand why those words had come to mind.

Suddenly my eyes were opened and I reflected back on an event from my early twenties when I had been a soda pop drinker. I had been listening to the radio that particular day when the host began talking about a study in a famous medical journal regarding the effects of caffeine in the body. I recalled my skin tingling and a sickly, anxious feeling churning in my belly as the commentator spoke. He said that a major ingredient in soda was caffeine and that it was added for its addictive properties. Nothing more. I was being exploited for profit. The queasiness in my stomach changed to anger. That day I resolved to quit drinking it—cold turkey.

Two days later I developed a chronic, splitting headache; was jittery; and grew impatient more quickly. I was sluggish and felt a strong pull to stop at the local mini-mart to fill my cup with fizzy cola comfort. It dragged on for weeks, and the lingering effects of the caffeine in my body sucked my energy dry. Then one day, it just stopped. My mind opened like an evening breeze had blown through and cleared everything undesirable out! Finally I could breathe.

My mind came back to the moment. I tossed my rag in the sink and walked to the pantry. My head flooded with years' of marketing tricks that I had been bombarded by, and I imagined how the pictures and clever jingles played into my own unhealthy-lifestyle decisions. I had always been annoyed by the excessiveness of TV commercials advertising everything under the sun. There were at least six pharmaceutical commercials on television in only one programming hour on any given day, and a dozen more inviting me to try some new fast food item. It was obvious manipulation by promotional ploy!

Opening the pantry door, I picked up a box and began reading the label. There were several ingredients I did not recognize and decided to type them into the computer and see what popped up. After doing so, my eyes grew large and my mouth dropped open. Tingling with anger, I learned the ingredients in question had been linked directly to cancer, not to mention a whole slew of other negative health problems—everything from heart disease to diabetes.

From that moment forward, instead of only reading about what was good for my body and how to heal it, I began searching for what was bad. It was a new facet of my gathering I had not yet fully explored. I had heard for years that certain ingredients were fine to ingest in "moderation," but I was waking up to the truth. I had only been lying to myself. Bad is bad no matter the amount.

Gaining a new resolve, I pulled the garbage can out from under the kitchen sink, slid it toward my pantry, and started waging war. Any label that reflected something mysterious was extricated. They landed in the garbage can with a liberating clunk. I threw out more than I kept.

It was then and there that I promised the Lord that I would take better care of my body for the rest of my life. A bizarre appreciation came over me regarding the cancer; without it, the years of studying the scriptures, or being open to learning new things, I would never have seen this truth—the truth that conspiring men actually wanted to make a buck off of my misfortune. Suddenly I was humbled and strangely grateful for contracting my illness. A warmth that felt a lot like the hot rays of the sun streaming through a south-facing window bathed me in satisfaction. I was learning.

Chapter Fourteen

GRATITUDE FOR CANCER

It was the end of September—seven-and-a-half months since I had met with Dr. Calder. The tumor had been growing since the biopsy. It discouraged me greatly and I cried about it a lot. I was doing everything I could to help myself, but instead of the anticipated result, the exact opposite was happening. The tumor was growing, pressing on my faith like a child repeating the phrase, "Are we there yet? Are we there yet?" Voices kept telling me that my faith was weak, and sometimes I believed it.

On occasion, my emotions sunk into a bottomless pit of despair and anger. I knew I was eating right. I was living *as if.* I was praying, I was reading the scriptures every day, and believed I was doing everything possible to heal; yet, there were no physical manifestations to that end. The experience was bringing with it a brutal torrent of cruel judgments directed towards me.

Too many times I missed the immediate promptings to pray more and instead suffered for hours ... and then Mike would come home. Poor Mike; I hardly gave him a chance to relax, pouncing on him the second he stepped into the house. I whined and cried about how horrible things were getting. He listened until I was finished, and then he would offer me a blessing.

Calm would once again cover me, and I quickly settled into a place of peace. Soon it became clear that as my faith grew there was an opposing force swelling proportionally. The paradigm provided a profound realization—life is like a pendulum; it swings one direction and then, invariably, must swing in the opposite direction. Just as Sir Isaac Newton had said, every action has "an equal and opposite reaction." I did not really like the idea that there had to be an opposing force but, indeed, there *had* to be; it was a law of nature.

As I recognized this pattern, the perception of my challenges changed. For each increase in my faith, Satan intensified his efforts to thwart my progress and everything would shift in the opposite direction. As my understanding grew, I came to know that it was going to happen and, of course, it did—again and again. However, I was better prepared for each round.

I wish I could say I never had another down day after recognizing the pattern, but that would not be true. There were still many difficult days. It was disheartening that I was unable to avoid days like this but, at least, while I was in the middle of them, I knew things would veer back the other direction … eventually. I wearied Mike with my incessant requests for blessings on those days.

When I felt particularly weak, I questioned my faith. Some days the darkness would come and suffocate me. More often, however I would receive a gentle nudge, reminding me to get back down on my knees and pray. Heavenly Father was teaching me to trust Him—implicitly.

During one of these instances, when I was in need of a blessing, Mike spoke a phrase that had so much power attached to it that it pervaded my attention for days afterward. He said, "Spiritual understanding is coming quicker to you than it would to others because of your struggles."

As strange as it may sound, that was the second time I was grateful for my cancer. Because of my experiences, spiritual rewards were creating a clear and solid connection between me and Jesus Christ. I was gaining an understanding of Him and what He had done for all mankind. I was learning how to let the atonement carry the burden, exactly as Steve had told me months before. I was learning to trust *His* process for my life.

Cancer was my cross to bear, but it was *nothing* in comparison to His. In a peculiar way, having cancer—and all I had gone through and what I was about to go through—emboldened me. Eventually, it would become an even greater blessing than my healing.

Chapter Fifteen

SLIDING OUT OF CONTROL

My greatest desire has always been to sing. As I continued to live as if nothing were wrong in my life, the Lord began opening many doors and I made numerous connections, which eventually led to being invited to sing with different orchestras in Utah. These connections were another manifestation of heavenly forces working in my life.

Relief filled my heart and I began to find a stronger sense of faith, and to feel powerful for more than just a few hours at a time. Joy exploded in my soul on a level I had never experienced before. For whatever reason, I was granted access to places I had always longed to be musically. It made it easier to move ahead with my dreams.

October arrived and the much-anticipated season of music was quickly coming together. I looked at the upcoming events as a distraction that would whisk me through all of the holidays in a rush of involvement, and keep me from thinking about more serious things. I just prayed that I could keep the pain controlled long enough.

By mid-October I was in a fair amount of discomfort but it was somewhat manageable with over-the-counter medication. I was not happy about having to take any medication, but I was grateful for it. Unfortunately, I did not know any other way to function without it. So, for the time being, my diet consisted of a steady stream of pain pills every three or four hours.

The Friday before Halloween I popped 600 mgs of ibuprofen an hour before a concert I was to perform at with the Salt Lake Pops Orchestra. I felt it kick in and was fairly confident I would be able to complete my performance. Nate, the conductor of the orchestra, had written one of the songs specifically for my voice. He had only given it to me a few days before. In addition to learning the melody, I had to write the lyrics for it—in Latin.

By the end of the evening I was drained. The pain had been kept at bay, but my energy was gone. It struck me that my vitality was starting to slip, but I quickly and quietly tucked my concern away as I interacted with the audience and signed a few autographs.

I made my way over to Mike who had been following me around with the camera.

"I'm wiped out," I said. "The pain is coming back."

He wrapped his arm around my shoulder and walked me toward the dressing room to collect my things. However, we were stopped by two other singers featured in the show.

"You were amazing!" Jen said enthusiastically, reaching out to touch my arm.

Nyrie chimed in, "Yes! Wow. That was incredible . . . those notes you hit . . . just wow!" The smile on her face told me everything I needed to know—the evening was a success.

I smiled and thanked them, responding in kind about their beautiful gifts. Mike suggested a photo or two, so we turned and smiled.

Afterward Jen turned and hugged me. I winced quietly. It was apparent that physical contact without pain medication in my system was now an issue. That was a new discovery.

"That was fun. I love you," she said.

"Thank you. I love you too!" I said with a smile as I squeezed her forearm.

Then Nyrie leaned in for a hug. I was prepared for her and kept a little more space between us. "Oh, you were just so amazing. Thank you for sharing your talents," she said exuberantly.

I smiled. Pain was beginning to double me over. Mike swooped in, took me by the waist and walked me backstage. I signaled an "I love you" in sign language to Nyrie as we left.

Stepping into the dressing room, we found my purse and I immediately began digging for the bottle of pills feeling like a junkie. When I located it, I began fighting with the lid. Mike took it from me and opened it, depositing three pills into my palm. He handed me a cup of water and I swallowed hard, and said a silent prayer. Mike slipped my coat around my shoulders and we walked out the back door. Leaving rather abruptly, I hoped no one had noticed anything odd.

~

By the end of November, the three-pill dosage of medication no longer covered the pain. Mike and I had talked about the frequency and dangers of taking drugs long-term. By that time I had increased them to 1,000 mg every three hours. I was mortified and scared. The worst part was, if I missed a dose, it would take about four hours to catch back up.

Life had gotten really busy. In addition to the multiple singing engagements, I was also recording an on-location music video and had several audio recording sessions. I was busy writing press releases for the local paper to promote two events in our small town, and trying to balance life at home. I had everything succinctly organized.

December hit, and just like a blizzard with white-out conditions, my life exploded into the moment-by-moment flurry of events I had created for myself. It kept me completely distracted from what was happening with my body, for which I was grateful.

I attempted to keep the pain contained and submissive to my insane calendar. The busyness of life kept me from thinking. In fact, when a negative thought would sneak to the surface, I would immediately bury it. I could not afford to think about the "what ifs" with the schedule I was keeping. Whatever climax was going to happen, I expected it after Christmas.

Early in the month of December, I noticed an area on the top of my breast was raised slightly, and over the next week it grew to the size of a quarter. I knew things had been changing, but I was unwavering in my decision to not go to a doctor. I knew what the suggestion would be and I knew I still would not take the advice.

One afternoon I became rather alarmed at the sight of the raised area and made a decision to call a friend of ours who was also a doctor. He was a member of our church and knew of my decision to go holistic, offering to help if I needed him at any point. It made me cringe to realize I was about to take him up on his offer.

I forced myself to dial his number. I almost hung up, but then I heard a pleasant female voice say, "Dr. Johnson's office, how can I help you?"

I stammered, "Oh, um, I'd like to schedule an appointment."

She asked for my name and then proceeded to schedule me in a few days later. I thanked her and hung up the phone. I felt angry and confused, and wondered if I had made the right decision.

~

The day of the appointment arrived and Mike and I stepped into the exam room. I was annoyed and certainly not happy to be there—especially because of embarrassment for the way my breast looked; it had grown red and angry looking, and I was ashamed to expose it to anyone, much less someone I knew from church.

In my head, giving in and going to a doctor translated as a deficit in my faith. I mentally worked to justify it; that it was only for information designed to help me understand what might be happening. I was resolute about staying away from treatment suggestions offered by the traditional medical industry.

One might think that under these circumstances I would have felt comforted that the doctor was someone we knew—someone who had a vested interest in my wellbeing. But I did not. I was suppressing incalculable levels of rage. I could feel it gurgling just under the surface, my face growing hot. No doubt the usual spotty redness was emblazoned across my chest.

A few minutes later, Dr. Johnson stepped in, smiling at both Mike and me. I returned an obligatory grin, but was not feeling it at all.

After detailing what was happening, he asked to see the area. Every cell in my body froze, making it difficult to even lie back on the table. Dr. Johnson placed one of his hands on my upper back, assisting me. The paper under my back crunched and crackled. His touch made me flinch and I wanted to scream. I shivered, holding the gown I had been given earlier like a protective shield. I had to force myself to release my grip on it when Dr. Johnson said, "May I?"

I watched his face intently as he pulled the gown back; nothing. No quail, no wince, no nothing. It took all of about fifteen seconds before he laid the gown back across my chest. Dr. Johnson had known us for years and was very aware that I was a modest person. He made every effort to help me feel that way, but it was not enough to erase my feelings of invasion.

I sat up. Dr. Johnson had taken a step back and said, "I'm really concerned about this; it looks like Inflammatory Breast Cancer."

I grimaced at the sound of it. It was ominous and big and from what I had already read about it; deadly. That was the worst possible comment he could have made.

He asked if I were willing to see a specialist. Internally I said, "No!" But outwardly, I agreed. I was in denial again about the possibilities. I refused to believe my cancer had developed into something lethal—that would be contrary to my previous validation from God—so it had to be, simply, some sort of liquid that needed draining. That is what I told myself.

Under circumstances such as these, I typically would have run the gamut of emotions—from terror, to anger, to fear—but not this time. Instead of disheartening words from the various articles I had read, which often gathered and screamed irreverently, something different happened; resolve took over. I could almost feel my heels dig in a little deeper. My calves even flexed. I was going to find a way out of this—just like the Lord had said I would. My faith was gaining strength.

~

That night I felt a little miffed and asked for a blessing. Mike agreed, of course. The comments were comforting. He said that I would "know" what needed to happen, that Heavenly Father was impressed with my faith and what I had done to show it, and that He would bless me for it. He said that the Lord was "pleased" with my giving this Christmas season, and that He was using me as a special tool in order to reach out to others.

Irritation left me and I felt myself crack a slight smile. The words from the blessing indicated that He wanted me to share my gift, and I was certain He would keep His promises.

Mike's voice increased in volume and fervor. He added, "You are on the correct path. Immerse yourself in the scriptures. Pray often. I bless you with the strength to accomplish your singing docket. Continue your consumption of nutrients. Heavenly Father knows you are doing the best you can. Ask for help."

The blessing finished and, as usual, I grabbed a pen and quickly jotted down what I remembered before it evaporated. The impressions were strong and gave me encouragement.

I found that I had been relying on the Lord more than ever, and my faith continued to develop as each new challenge arrived. This confidence in God would become the anchor that held me secure through the storms that were coming. Breathing in, I began scribbling again.

When I finished, I looked over my schedule. There was a week-and-a-half until I would meet with the specialist, which would be the sixteenth of the month—right in the middle of everything in which I was involved. I was grateful it was December and that I was busy so I did not have down time to stew about it.

Chapter Sixteen

EVEN IF I DIE

The appointment day with the specialist arrived. Even though it had been ten months since I had received the diagnosis from Dr. Calder, her remarks were still very fresh in my mind and I was not interested in undergoing another emotional assault from this new doctor. I only sought clarification. I geared up my mind for the meeting.

It concerned me that I could potentially fold under the pressure again so I prayed for strength, and mentally readied myself for the appointment; I only wanted information. As I checked in with the front desk, I elongated my neck in an attempt to feel more authoritative.

On the outside I was dressed sharply, poised and full of confidence. With my heels, I was nearly six-feet tall, providing, what I thought to be, an intellectual and visual advantage. On the inside, however, my nerves were taught, about ready to slip over the edge. I could feel Satan banging on the back door of my brain, hoping I would crack it open just enough for him to get a toe in, and then I realized he was already in. That played right into the same emotion I experienced during the very first ultrasound appointment. In frustration, I let out an exasperated sound from my mouth, but at least this time I had an awareness of his presence and began working to remove him.

"Oh, no you don't!" I said, "You're not welcome here."

I closed my eyes, rolling them; shook my head and inhaled, filling my lungs with air.

"You're going to be just fine, and no one is going to take away your power. You're the only one who can give it away," I thought to myself.

I sat up straight and purposefully imagined myself being filled with strength. Just then a nurse called my name. I stood, squared my shoulders, and then followed her into the back.

We walked into the tiny exam room. I thought it seemed odd that the ceiling rose higher than the actual square footage of the floor. There was a small stainless-steel sink; one set of drab, peachy-colored cupboards; a built-in desk; and a small, black stool.

The nurse reached into a drawer on the side of the exam table and laid a thin, white paper sheet on the top, which was neatly folded. Then she asked that I undress from the waist up and cover myself with the sheet. When she shut the door, I lifted the sheet up to the light.

"Not much to it, is there?" I said aloud to myself.

It reminded me of the paper towels under my kitchen sink, except this was even thinner.

"I should have brought my own," I thought. "It would have had more substance."

A few minutes later, Dr. Howard came in, followed by a slender, red-haired nurse. He had a neatly-trimmed, full scalp of dark-brown hair and deep-set, cinnamon-colored eyes.

He seemed pleasant. The thought blazed through my mind that I was sitting there with a complete stranger, half-dressed, with only a sheer paper towel between us. Internally, I squirmed uncomfortably. Feelings of being violated saturated me again and a shiver ran down my back. A dense, unseen haze began creeping in, pressing down on me. I tried to shake it and act as though nothing bothered me. I reasoned that my bareness was nothing to a doctor. He had likely seen plenty of bodies every day of his career; but for me, it was far too revealing.

After a few moments of awkward, idle conversation, he asked me to lie back on the exam table. The paper table covering crackled under my body. The sound now represented something negative and irritation flooded in.

Dr. Howard was surprisingly conscientious about not exposing too much of my body. That helped me relax. As he examined me, I caught myself nervously talking, telling him what I thought was going on.

"I think it's filled with liquid," I said, trying not to sound as nervous as I felt.

He said, "What are your expectations of me today?"

"To lance the bump and drain it," I said, sure of my own diagnosis.

He acknowledged my comment and turned to the nurse, whose name badge twisted just enough for me to see her name was McKayla. He told her what instruments to get from the cupboard, which she promptly did. Thankfully, he covered my skin while he waited.

When the nurse gave him a syringe he turned, uncovered me and pierced the bump. And then it hit me.

"What if it isn't liquid? What if it's actually the tumor and he was potentially spreading the cancer cells throughout my body?" I screamed at myself. "Alicia! You did it again! What is wrong with you?"

I froze, listening intently to the inundation of abuses I was heaping on myself. I was immediately cold, and a black shadow cloaked my brain in dread. I wondered how I got there, how I had so easily slipped right back to a place where I had no restraint. "Why would I even ask him to lance the thing?" I closed my eyes and they rolled backward.

Alarm shot through me. After studying everything I had about what a biopsy could potentially mean to the growth of a tumor, what was I thinking? I clenched my teeth and dug my fingernails into the sides of the table, searching for answers. I could feel my knuckles turning white. Blood drained from my face. I was incredulous at my shortsighted thinking. A shiver was getting ready to erupt, but I caught it, shoving it to the back of my body. I was not about to tip my hand to Dr. Howard.

Forcing my hands to let go of the table, I commanded my body to relax. I created an imaginary bulldozer that shoved everything out, and then I refocused and tried to call on God. At first the words I thought of were angry and full of condemnation, but then I stopped myself. As I gathered my wits, I started again, asking for peace and the ability to remember my direction; the direction I had received from Him.

Slowly I began to feel warmer, and a strong sense of acceptance flooded over me. I was about to acknowledge it and thank the Lord for it but Dr. Howard spoke, interrupting my prayer. "There is no liquid inside. It's only tissue." He gave the nurse the needle, and pulled the sheet to my shoulder. His demeanor changed, almost on a dime. His eyes grew dark and his white teeth barely showed behind the tight line of his lips.

"You need to see an oncologist," he said, as he helped me sit upright.

I looked at him, wondering why his manner had shifted so significantly, and felt my resolve weakening.

"I'm not interested in doing that," I said more feebly than I wanted.

He did not react to my remark, but looked down at his hands and removed his gloves. Then he turned his back and moved toward the door, saying, "I'm going to step out for a moment so you can get dressed, and then I'll come back and we'll talk." He opened the door for the nurse who gave him a knowing glance, and then they exited rather quickly.

The glance burned. What was she thinking? I climbed off the exam table and dressed as fast as possible, preparing to contest the statement the doctor had just made. I squeezed my eyes shut, and prayed for direction as I pulled my shirt on, and tucked it in.

I continued my prayer. The powers of heaven slowly began pouring down upon me and my confidence came back in full force. I threw my shoulders back and stood tall in my heels. The earlier fog I had sensed lifted and I felt strong and unyielding again.

My course was already set and I knew it. There was no need to question it, or even see another doctor. The Lord had already told me I was going to live and that I needed to follow my heart. My determination expanded to a new height. Determination and certainty settled over me about the path I was on. I sat down on a chair, closed my eyes, and breathed in and out slowly—letting the assurance soak in completely.

"It's your body; you can do whatever you want," I repeated to myself, as Mike's freedom-giving words replayed inside of me. I was filled with assurance and gratitude.

A few minutes later Dr. Howard knocked and then stepped back into the room, closing the door behind him. He was alone this time.

He looked at his hands, which he rubbed together slowly. He said, "What do you want to do?" After a moment of silence, he looked up at me. There was an obvious wrinkle in my brow. He already knew the answer to the question.

"Are you willing to speak to an oncologist?" he asked in a fairly severe manner. "There are two right across the hall and there is an opening tomorrow."

I chuckled inward, and took exception to his parental tone. A sense of incredulity began to spread within me, "Not now," I stated firmly.

"I've read the notes in your chart from Dr. Calder." he said, looking at his feet first and then directly at me.

My understanding of the earlier change in his behavior sunk in. I thought, "Ah, that's why you are being so forceful. You read my chart from Dr. Calder and you see that I never responded to her requests for treatment."

He continued, "When you were diagnosed, the tumor was the size of a key lime, now it's as big as an orange." His tone lifted in pitch and came across as quite reckless. He was pushing the issue with me and using scare tactics to boot. He pointed out the obvious; I knew how large the tumor had grown. His change in conduct and his uncaring insistence did not bode well with me, and I wondered why he was forcing the issue.

He persisted, "I put you on a list to talk to one of the oncologists."

I have no doubt the look of surprise on my face struck Dr. Howard. I felt my eyebrows lift. "I'm sorry, what? You put me on a list?" My voice sounded irritated. "You need to take me off that list. I'm not doing that." I was almost shocked at the strength with which I made the statement. The powers of heaven were driving my conviction. I took heart in that.

I was screaming at him, but he heard nothing vocalized. "How dare you! Who do you think you are? You are not going to force me to do something I have not authorized. You will not decide what course of action I will take!"

I stared at him in disbelief that he would do such a thing without my consent. I had already said no. He knew that, yet still attempted to shove me in a direction I did not wish to go. He was trying to take away my power. He purposefully tapped into my fear, which solidified my determination that he was the last person on the planet I would listen to since he was unwilling to listen to me.

His appearance changed and he darkened even more than before. His brow crumpled, and the corners of his mouth drooped into a frown. "You ... need ... to ... meet ... with ... an ... oncologist," he said, clenching his teeth slightly and accentuating each word as if they were singular. "You need chemotherapy and radiation immediately. It's the *only* course to take."

The look on his face caused me to dig in even deeper and the tension in the room rose sharply. He was attempting to constrain me.

"Coercion is not the Lord's way," I thought as confidence fused itself into my body again.

If this was the doctor's idea of attempting to sell me on the idea of seeing an oncologist, it was not working. I was grateful for my experiences with Dr. Calder. Both of them had taught me something. Although the medical route was the "only course of action to take" for some people, it certainly was not the *only* course. What resonated with me, however, was something more. This clinic, and thousands more just like it, were not only a place where patients came to seek help for their medical problems, it was also a business. Dr. Howard's intention may have been to help me, but his approach sent a different message.

Refusing his push, I took a deep breath, knowing that I was awake and aware now, and attended by the Lord. I could feel Him swell in my heart, giving me courage to push back. I sat up straight and lowered my chin, focusing intently on his eyes.

"I don't intend to do that," I said firmly.

His eyes sparked. "Even if you die?" He asked boldly, training his focus on me.

I expect that he did, in fact, expect me to die. I almost laughed at his audacity.

My gaze did not falter and inwardly I said, "Yes, even if I die. Besides, who are you to even suggest such a thing? There is only one person who can decide when I die, and it's not you!" I felt a little smug again. Nothing audible came out of my mouth though.

I did not fear Dr. Howard. In fact, his remark about dying did not frighten me at all. Suddenly and fully, I knew the Lord had other plans for me. I rehearsed my mantra: The doctor did not love me, nor did he care for me, which was apparent from his behavior. Whatever his agenda was, I was not participating in it today. I was not afraid anymore. I dismissed him from the room, put on my coat and left his office.

I smiled to myself, raised my hand and simulated a flick with my finger, representing Dr. Howard's ejection from what I came to call my life list. He was no longer worthy to be on it. In my current vein of thinking, only those with positive attitudes and encouraging language were allowed admittance into my life, even if it meant death—but it did not. I was assured of that by the sweet whisperings of the Holy Spirit.

As I walked toward my car, I thought about what most other people would have done under similar conditions; they would likely have agreed to his suggestions. I was a rebel, being driven by my faith and trust in Heavenly Father. Feelings of liberation infused me, and I realized the seeds I had planted so many months ago were now a sturdy little tree with roots sinking deep into the ground. I knew the Lord had stood by my side and had given me mighty strength—that which was beyond my own—allowing me to act in a way that exceeded my own abilities.

So, with the exception of Dr. Howard's declaration about the contents of the bump, I possessed no more information than I had before I met him, and, in addition, expected a $300 bill for the experience. I grasped the best part of the entire situation—the Lord had given me sureness and certitude; thus, the experience was worth every nickel.

Leaving the office parking area, I drove to the location where I was scheduled to sing that afternoon. Twenty-four hours prior I was unsure whether I would even be in the mood. But now I was almost giddy. It was going to be a strong performance.

~

The rest of December went by in a veritable haze. My insane performance schedule drove me. How I loved singing and sharing the gifts I had been given! For now, the pain was being managed most of the time. Peace filled my life. It seemed strange to me, but it also made sense; the Lord was fulfilling His promises.

There was one thing looming however; when Christmas was over, then what? I sensed a change was coming, and it made me nervous.

Chapter Seventeen

THE SEASON OF GIVING

Ten and a half months had passed since I had met with Cowboy Don, but one morning I awoke with him on my mind. I tried to shake it, but it kept popping in. I thought to call him, but I kept shoving the idea out. It scared me for some reason. But the notion would not leave.

Don and I had texted back and forth frequently throughout that year. I would update him on my condition and ask questions, but we had never actually spoken by phone. He always seemed interested, and I felt confident that he would be willing to speak to me.

It had been a little over a month since I had texted him, and while I was nervous, I was also excited that I was brave enough to consider the idea. When I located his number in my cell phone's address book, I pressed dial. It rang twice, and then I heard a recording say, "I'm sorry, the number you have dialed has been disconnected."

My heart dropped! "Oh no!" For a few minutes panic seized me. Almost as quickly, things shifted and I calmed, remembering that I also had his home phone number. I let out a sigh and breathed deeply, trying to slow my heartbeat.

When the adrenaline stopped speeding through my veins, I began to consider what I would say to Don, and why I was even calling him. I looked at his home phone number. Bothering him while he was with family disturbed me. It felt like the call, if made, would be an intrusion into his private life and I did not want to take advantage of his kindness. But intuition kept tapping on my forehead, so after contemplating it for a time, I called. Don's son answered. I told him who I was and that I had tried calling his dad, but that his cell phone number wasn't working.

He said, "Oh yeah. He got a new number because so many people were trying to get free consultations out of him."

It was a good thing we weren't face to face, because I could feel an immediate flush of red hit my face; my reasons were the same. I needed to consult with Don and I had no money. I almost said something to the young man about it but, instead, froze and bit my tongue.

He continued, "Dad is in Australia, but he'll be back in two days."

I knew Don traveled frequently for business, but I was still disappointed that he was not available. It had taken quite a bit of courage to dial the number, and now I had to wait.

I inquired, "Would you mind taking my number and asking him to call me when he gets back into town?"

"Not at all," he said jovially.

"If he doesn't call me in three days, I'll try him in four or five," I replied.

"Okay, great," he responded.

I gave him my phone number, thanked him, and hung up the phone.

Laying the phone on the kitchen counter and shaking my head, I wondered if Don would be annoyed that I tracked him down at home … and for free information. The thoughts that forced themselves on me at that time were rude and sharp. There was not enough money to cover my current grocery bill, let alone pay for Don's expertise, but I was pretty desperate and motivated. I spent a few hours criticizing myself.

Eventually I came to the decision that Don would either answer my questions freely based on our limited friendship or he would establish a financial expectation right up front. Calmness filled me, and I knew whatever happened, the Lord was still influencing the outcome.

Five days passed and no call from Don ... and I did not call him either. I was still a little hesitant about asking for free help. After nearly two weeks, I was getting anxious. The raised area on my breast was still growing, and the top layer was pulling tighter and tighter every day until small flakes of skin began to peel away from it. Although I was sure of the outcome of this journey, the fact remained—I did not know how far down I would have to go before I would come back up. That unknown scared me—regardless of my knowledge.

~

On December 23, I had my final concert of the season at our local mall. A sizeable group had gathered near the stage. The corridors and stores were filled with hundreds of last-minute shoppers. All the available seats were filled and the security detail rushed back and forth trying to tie up the loose ends. I smiled at Mom and Dad from the backside of the stage. They had driven down from Boise and arrived early to claim their seats, front and center. All of my kids came, and some of my friends, too. There was a tangible excitement in the air.

Lifting my long, shimmery red skirt away from my feet, I climbed up the stairs and onto the stage. Shoppers paused, their arms loaded with bags of holiday presents. Little girls jumped up and down and pointed, squealing loudly until their mothers noticed what they were excited about. Then everything stopped and a hush fell over the crowd. I was the center of attention, surrounded by people on all sides of the platform.

I introduced myself and thanked everyone for coming, and then motioned to my daughter Jill, who was running the sound equipment. The music filled the hallways with the sweet strains of Christmas music. For over an hour I shared my love of Christ through song.

When the final number had been presented, the little girls began bouncing again, yanking on the arms of whomever was closest until they were escorted to where I was standing. Numerous little girls, and even a little boy or two, stood before me with bright eyes and big smiles. Their loud, excited voices immediately dropped to near silence and they batted their eyes shyly. As I spoke to them one by one, the crowd dissipated and I turned my attention to my parents.

Several minutes later I became aware that someone else was tugging on my skirt. I looked down; a darling, blue-eyed, blonde- and curly-haired girl of the tiniest stature stood there. She was about five or six and was wearing a white coat with a pale fur collar. She smiled widely. I smiled back, squatted down next to her and said, "Hi there! What's your name?"

"Grace," she said, wide-eyed, and then exclaimed, "You are beautiful!"

I chuckled. "Thank you, Grace, but I think you are the beautiful one."

She stared at me for a long time without blinking or speaking. All I could do was hold her hands in mine and smile back. I remembered being just like her when I was little—wide-eyed and awestruck by someone in a princess dress. I was just as mesmerized by her as she seemed to be with me. Then a thought hit me and I realized I held a tiny piece of her future in the palm of my hands, and whatever I chose to say to her could potentially impact her forever.

I asked, "Do you like to sing, Grace?"

She nodded enthusiastically without speaking, but I could see in her eyes that it was something she loved.

"Well then, Grace, no matter what, you must sing! If you love it, you must sing every day. Practice all the time and when you grow up you can bring a lot of happiness to people when they hear your voice," I said to her.

You might have thought it was Christmas morning by the look in her twinkling, animated eyes. "I will!" she said eagerly. "Thank you for singing tonight. It was so beautiful."

"You're welcome pretty girl! Have a Merry Christmas!" I said as she turned to walk away, and then all at once she spun back toward me, ran into my arms and hugged my neck tightly.

"Thank you!" she exclaimed.

She turned again and leaped a few steps forward into the arms of her mother, who locked on and mouthed the words, "Thank you." There was a tear in her eye.

A spirit of joy washed over me, nearly bringing me to tears. I choked and held my breath as they pushed through the crowd and disappeared. That was a good night. It reminded me exactly what Christmas is all about—love and service. If my gift touched a mother and her daughter so deeply, then it was worth the hours of rehearsals in order to share that gift with them.

I quietly said a prayer, grateful that I had been allowed to bless the life of that little girl. I knew without question the warmth of the holidays was exactly what Grace needed to feel that night. It was a gift from the Savior that had passed through me to her. I took great satisfaction in that. My own personal courage rose, knowing that if I were able to affect a little girl in such a special way, surely the Lord would continue to bless me through other people as well.

I will never know the impact I had on that beautiful little girl that night, but her mother's emotion lingered with me for days afterward.

~

The next night was Christmas Eve and our annual family party. I had been looking forward to it for months. The feverish energy of my hectic performance schedule mellowed into a sweet and peaceful calm that permeated my house like the scented candle I had lit. It felt good to slow down and focus my attentions on family.

The house smelled wonderful and the Christmas tree shone bright and beautiful in the corner, its blue lights glowing—just like the moonlit snow outside my window. I surveyed the room. The presents were wrapped and tucked under the tree, a few extra chairs had been placed in the living room, and the fireplace was ablaze, warming every corner.

One by one the kids arrived. Mom and Dad were already there, and Mike had driven over the mountain to pick up his father to bring him to our

91

celebration, too. It did not take long before the room was bursting at the seams and filled with laughter.

In the hustle and bustle, I did not hear the alarm on my phone go off. I had it set to ring every three hours as a reminder to take my painkillers. An hour later, I felt the twinge of pain coming on. I gasped, putting my hand to my mouth and called myself "stupid."

Trying not to alert anyone, I quickly and quietly grabbed five pills and swallowed them with a glass of water. I was so angry, and whispered to Mike, "Of all days to miss a dose," I said with a whimper in my voice.

"It'll be all right," he said in my ear, trying to comfort me.

It did not take long for the pain to develop into a serious distraction for me. It radiated on the side of my breast and began throbbing unforgivingly, making it difficult to breath or focus. I caught myself leaving the room from time to time, trying to deal with it. But since there was a house full of guests, I was forced to press on. With each passing minute, the pain grew more intense. I prayed and prayed that I would be able to finish the evening without grimacing too much.

Four hours later, the pain began to subside. We were right in the middle of opening presents when I started functioning on a clearer level. No one, with the exception of Mike, had been the wiser because there was so much activity going on. It hit me that the pain had multiplied greatly since the last time I had missed a dose. That scared me. It was an indication that things were still under constant progression, and a reminder that my full attention would have to shift after Christmas.

Chapter Eighteen

AND SO IT BEGINS

A few days later it was Sunday and the bishop from our church called both Mike and me into his office. I fully intended to keep my cancer problem to myself, but somehow the conversation went in an unexpected direction and I found myself opening up and telling him. Mike looked at me oddly, knowing that my aim was to remain silent about it. I shrugged my eyebrows at him feeling a little vulnerable at my brash admission.

The bishop looked shocked. Inside I could feel myself shudder at the fact that his jaw was hanging open. It never ceased to amaze me—the reactions from unsuspecting listeners. I stared at him, trying not to let it affect me. He stumbled over his words, and then composed himself.

"Do you have insurance?" he asked softly.

I felt grateful that he did not share any cancer stories with us; that was unusual for someone on the outside.

Mike spoke, which woke me out of my trance. "We have some, but it will be canceled at the end of the year."

"Then what are you going to do?" The bishop asked.

Mike looked over at me, then back to the bishop. "I guess we won't have any."

The bishop looked a little concerned and made a few suggestions, stating that we "might need it" at some future point, and he suggested that we look into it.

I could not fathom needing it; I fully expected to heal. I expected the Lord to do his part, because I was doing mine. Mike, however, took it as a prompting to at least see if there were something out there for a preexisting condition that would not break the bank.

As we left the office, a strange feeling wrapped around my body, and I thought I might throw up. It was a silent battle between the faith I was trying to maintain and weakness, which shuffled in by the unruly thought of insurance. Once again, the unwelcome word "procedure" slipped in.

~

Although we had not spent a dime of it yet, Mom and Dad had given us some money for Christmas three weeks prior to the actual holiday. We had so many needs that it was difficult to decide where to put it. Finally, after deliberating for a few weeks, I told Mike about some products I wanted to order, which were supposed to help with self-healing. The only problem was, my prayers regarding them were met with impressions of indecision and hesitancy. That should have been my answer, but the written declarations from other users were so definitive that I gave in to my own feelings and ignored the spiritual ones.

A few days after Christmas the products arrived—eight small bottles with eyedroppers for lids. The instructions were simple enough; add six drops to a cup and drink them morning and evening. At first I did not notice anything different, but as the substance began building up in my system, things changed rapidly.

My level of energy plunged. I would get up in the morning feeling fine, leave the house to take on the day, and then hit an imaginary brick wall a few hours later, which caused me to change all of my plans and hurry back home where I would fall asleep. Then, I would wake up three or four hours later, eat dinner with Mike, and go to bed—hours before my normal bedtime. Whatever was going on, it was quickly taking over and stealing my energy. For a time, I thought my body was simply going through a detox stage, and that it would get worse before it got better. It did not take long before I was convinced that my rational was incorrect.

On January 3, I got dressed and went to my part-time job. I had only been there for a few hours when I realized I was not going to make it through the rest of the day, so I called in a replacement.

I barely made it home. I fell onto the couch and slept for five hours. When I awoke, I knew something was very wrong with me. I prayed, and then realized the answer I was seeking had already been given me. I decided to quit the liquids immediately. That decision was coupled with a feeling of peace and comfort, as though I had finally gotten back onto the track the Lord intended for me. Then the words to a scripture came to mind. *"For God is not the author of confusion, but of peace …"* (1 Corinthians 14:33; KJV; emphasis added).

I censured myself. "What is wrong with you, Alicia? As if you didn't have enough to deal with, you do this to yourself! You need to pay closer attention to the promptings you feel and stop trying to do it alone."

For the next hour I fell into a dark place. Satan knew I was angry with myself for not listening to the Lord, and he pounded that thought deeper and deeper into me like a railroad spike. It pierced my head and chest, and the weight of it grew heavier and heavier, until I could barely breathe. Darkness shrouded me and put me in a place of fear and dread, which I had avoided for many weeks. It was as though someone had shoved me into a pit filled with cold, muddy water. My body squirmed and my skin crawled, feeling like a thousand spiders were crawling across it. For a while I was completely blind to any light at all. Satan might as well have been right there, screaming at me; maybe he was.

When Mike came in, he found me rolled up in a ball, crying.

"Oh, Alicia!" He said in a tone that expressed two things—sorrow and dismay. I knew him well enough to know that my pain was his. I also knew it was wearing him out.

I was in a seated position on the couch with my arms wrapped tight around my knees. Mike hurried to my side, pulling me to his. It shook me loose from Satan's grip, and suddenly without a lot of warning, that familiar wrenching sound burst from my lips and split the air. My body heaved and sobbed and shook. Mike drew me in closer, holding me increasingly tighter.

My body convulsed for what felt like twenty minutes. I let go of my knees and my hands fell loose, landing on Mike's lap with a soft thud. I could feel the evil seeping from every corner of my body. The heaviness of my breathing and the whimpering sounds that accompanied it began to quiet, and soon I found myself melding into Mike's body.

Slowly I gained restraint over the darkness that had permeated the room but it did not completely dissipate. My sobs were slowing and I heard myself say, "I can feel myself going down. My body is failing!"

I did not share my views with Mike at the time, but I asked myself, "What if this seemingly simple act of unintended disobedience causes me to be unworthy of being healed? What if I die because of it?" The declarations were loud and prevalent, and draped over me in penetrating black tones.

I was frenzied when Mike whispered, "I'll be right here, no matter what."

His words swirled around me in a symphony of white light that chased away every fiber of evil that had previously been there. I repeated his words several times, allowing them to comfort me. I cried again. Mike leaned his cheek against my hair, trying to lift my burdens and carry them away from me. But it was no longer an affliction; instead, it was gratitude that fused itself into me. I knew the Lord had heard my silent plea and that He was going to heal me.

Chapter Nineteen

FARMA, NOT PHARMA

Christmas was barely a week behind me and, as predicted, the change I had sensed came in hard and fast. I was on massive amounts of medication—forty pills in a typical twenty-four-hour period. The pills were not keeping the discomfort in check anymore and eight thousand milligrams of Ibuprofen a day frightened me; I knew the level was too high, but the agony I was in superseded any logic I may have had.

The pain came in waves; it ebbed for a while and then would wash in, in typhoon style, knocking me to my knees—figuratively and literally. The continued swelling was causing awkwardness in my movements and I could not take a step without putting an arm across my chest as a brace. Any type of jarring would fold me over in pain.

Physically I felt whipped. I was sleep deprived, waking up every three hours to take more pills, and I was over-sleeping during the day, trying to catch up with the nocturnal losses. With zero energy, cooking had become a thing of the past because I could not stand long enough to prepare anything. I did not even have the stamina to juice anymore, which made me feel like I had fallen below the nutritional level I had established for myself. It was all I could do to walk the ten paces to the kitchen to get an apple or some nuts. Often I just went without. I did not notice any hunger, only weight loss. My yoga pants began to hang on me. I felt like everything I had been doing was being ruined by my inability to continue caring for myself properly, which made me wonder if the cancer would take over and kill me anyway.

As the elevated area on my breast continued to rise, the skin pulled tighter and peeled away like badly sunburned skin. I did not know whether to panic or endure quietly. It was like climbing a large mountain where the peak was masked by clouds, and I had no idea where the top was. My faith was still strong, but there were definite lapses in my confidence. It happened so often, in fact, that I questioned the echelon of my faith almost daily.

One evening after I had taken a bath and was getting ready for bed, I examined the bump. The skin was still flaking. I reached up and pulled off a fragment that was hanging on by mere fibers. Abruptly, blood began draining from the area. That minute piece of flesh was the only thing holding back the steady, thin stream that was now flowing from my chest into the bathroom sink. Mike was downstairs and I called for him in a tone that probably scared him because he moved up the stairs faster than he ever had previously.

"What is it?" he asked before he had even reached the door. Then he stepped inside. His eyes grew wide. "Whoa, what happened?"

I am certain it was quite a sight. I was leaning over the sink as far as I could so the blood would not get onto my clothes or the floor.

"I just peeled a tiny piece of skin off, and it just started bleeding. There was hardly anything holding it back!" My voice was distressed and spinning with confusion.

Mike said, "I wonder if it's old blood. It looks dark."

I was impressed that his tone lacked emotion and was quiet and ordered. It made me feel better, and calmed the frenzied feeling I was experiencing.

"Maybe," I said. "That would make sense. It's been getting bigger the last few weeks, and my skin has been redder than before."

He suggested I watch it for a few minutes to see if the drainage slowed down. It did and I figured he was right about it being old blood because the overall tightness of my skin seemed to ease. That was actually a welcomed relief. I grabbed a towel, just in case, and headed into the bedroom. Mike had changed and was already in bed as I climbed between the covers, tucking the horde of pillows I had accumulated around my body to help with the ever present pain.

"Are you okay?" Mike asked, leaning up on one elbow.

"Yes," I responded, pausing to reflect on what had just happened. "That was weird. I don't know what to think about it," I said, as I grabbed an extra pillow and threw it to the floor.

"I think you'll be okay," he stated with a quiet, cool inflection in his voice. "If it had been something to worry about, I think it would have bled more. Don't you?" he asked in a voice that told me he really was not sure of the answer.

I shrugged, "Boy, I hope so."

Rolling over, I fell fast asleep, only to wake up three hours later to take part in my usual nighttime pill-popping ritual. There were no more blood issues that night.

~

The next morning everything seemed *normal*—if you want to call it that. Mike had left for work and I got out of bed, pulled on my yoga pants, and cautiously crept down the stairs to the kitchen, careful not to allow any movement that might jar my body. I felt a little lightheaded but, overall, I felt okay. I grabbed an apple and sat down on the couch.

Lying on the coffee table were my scriptures. I picked them up and began reading in Mark about Jesus. I had been studying His life on and off for over a year. It had become encouraging to me to read of the multiple miracles Christ performed on people—healing them. On this particular day I ran across a verse that had not really impacted me before, but this time it jumped off the page as though I were supposed to read it.

And a certain woman, which had *an issue of blood* twelve years,
and *had suffered many things of many physicians,* and had *spent all that*

99

she had, and was nothing bettered, but rather grew worse, when she heard of Jesus, came in the press behind, and touched his garment. For *if I may touch but his clothes, I shall be whole. And straightway the fountain of her blood was dried up*; and she felt in her body that *she was healed* of that plague (Mark 5: 25-29; KJV; emphasis added).

I could relate to that woman. My experience with doctors to this point was similar, and I had not been healed yet. I needed a robe to touch.

It was clear the Lord was trying to tell me something. The woman's trust was in Him—*not in men*—and that was what healed her. I prayed that He would open the door of my understanding and help me see what else I needed to do so that I, like her, might be healed. As usual, He answered that prayer.

~

January 5 was a Saturday. It had been around two weeks since I had spoken to Don Tolman's son on the phone. I was a bit frustrated about that and promised myself I would call him Monday morning, which would be a workday. I did not want to disrupt Don's family time. It was a precious commodity since his business frequently took him out of the country.

No more than five minutes later, the phone rang; it was Don. The impact was profound and I understood that I was being shown the next step to take. I did not think it was a coincidence that he called just then. As strange as it may sound, I trusted Don immediately because of that spiritual impression. Before I answered the call, I knew that whatever he suggested, I would do.

"Hello?" I said, trying to sound livelier than I felt.

"Hey, this is Cowboy Don," he said with a smile on his voice. "How are you doing?"

I hesitated. "A bit rough," I said, pausing again.

"Tell me what's been going on," he encouraged.

In many ways it was hard for me to let go of my voluntary, protective mentality. I closed my eyes tight and allowed the spirit of heaven to work on me, and to give myself permission to open the door. Then, as if I were a puppet suddenly animated by an invisible hand, I spilled everything to Don; how much medication I was currently taking, and how the raised area had bled a few days before, how my diet had become nonexistent, the weight loss, the increase in discomfort and how it was so hard to do anything because my energy was gone. I tried not to sound too much like a whiner, but I probably did. I just felt so overwhelmed by what seemed like rapid changes. Don listened quietly. It lifted the anvil off my shoulders as I shared my challenges with someone whom I felt had the answers I was searching for.

As he spoke, I wrote feverishly—trying to capture everything he said.

"The less you do, the less you can do. Life is movement. Restoring the electrical function to your body is critical. Walk twenty to thirty minutes a day, and if you don't have the strength to do that, walk a few minutes, and then add more over the course of a few days or weeks. Do what you're capable of." He stopped briefly and then said, "You have to be mentally strong. Your brain is in charge."

I thought of The Law of the Harvest as he was speaking, and was almost out of breath just listening to him. He was speaking at a lively pace, and I was writing as fast as I could. I did not want to miss a single word. My intention was to follow every instruction he detailed.

He paused so I interjected a question, "What about the Ibuprofen I'm taking?" I asked.

"Pills are *poisons*. They toxify the body. They don't heal and they *never* repair anything. If we're going to work together, you have to commit to changing those things. No pills. No capsules. No injections. No supplements of any kind. You have to support the nature of your own self-healing. Stop all of the poisoning and stressing of the body. Even though 'it's been proven,'" he said with a nasally tone, revealing to me his disdain for medical things, "it's not true—no pill or capsule is good for the body. Nature is not broken, we are!" he stated emphatically.

I knew I had to quit the pills, but my mouth dropped open anyway. How was I going to manage the pain if I stopped? For all my studying, I had not researched my medication of choice. I already had an opinion about them; they were bad for me, but I had not grasped that it would hinder my healing process until that very moment. How did I expect my body to win this fight if I kept feeding it chemicals that were in obvious conflict to the perfectly functioning immune system I sought? I was doing everything else right with my diet, but I had not even considered the effects of the pills. I had been careless. I committed right then and there to quit taking them.

Don continued. "It doesn't surprise me that you're so tired all the time. Five pills every three hours would put down a horse."

Although Don was not calling me out, I felt ashamed. Tears sprang to my eyes. I wiped them as they rolled down my cheeks and worked to keep the tipping of my emotions level. I did not like taking the meds, but I had been grateful for them, and I did not know any other way of combatting the pain. The thought of removing them scared me.

He continued, "Pharmaceuticals or any over-the-counter medications can actually cause pain. Did you know that pharm, as in pharmaceutical or pharmacy means poison maker or sorcery?" He paused temporarily. "True story; you can look it up online."

My mouth dropped open a little and I heard myself gasp. I wrote what he said on my paper. My intention was to look that information up as soon as I got off the phone. I was no scholar and knew very little about the root of most words, but what Don was telling me was creating a strange kind of order for me— as though I already knew.

Don talked about more things regarding pain management and the blood I had lost. He explained that it was a broken capillary and that he had known others who had experienced the same sort of thing. He seemed unemotional about it, which helped me feel less anxious. I concluded that the vein must have been leaking for a while and filled my breast with blood. I reasoned that it had been a good thing to let it drain as I had. Misguided thinking I came to regret later.

As he continued, Don talked about my diet, or lack thereof. He said, "What does a dog or a cat do when they're sick?"

Silence …. I did not know what to say.

"They do one of two things; they either stop eating all together or they eat grass until they throw up. They know what to do instinctively. Don't worry about the weight loss; it's your body's way of helping you heal," he said.

He sounded so sure of the information he was sharing that I did not question it. It sounded perfectly reasonable and I believed him.

The call ended and I turned to my notes. Noticing that I had written the word pharma on my pad, I pulled my computer to my lap and began searching the root word for it. Sure enough, what he said was accurate. It fed the fire I already had burning about prescriptions and medications, solidifying it. I was going to trust the Lord more and men less. I admit though, I was still afraid to quit taking my medication.

Chapter Twenty

AN ISSUE OF BLOOD

My alarm went off at three a.m. as usual. I carefully moved one of my pillows to the floor and pushed myself up, blinking to clear my eyes and acclimate to the darkness. There was a slight glow filtering in from the window that lit the room. I stood and went into the bathroom.

After I had closed the door, I felt something strange and warm on my chest. I reached over, fumbling for the switch on the nightlight, and flipped it on. I was bleeding! I stared in disbelief as the stain on my shirt quickly spread like a spigot had been turned on. Quickly I ripped off my shirt, careful not to drag it across my face or hair. By the time it was safely clutched between both hands in front of me, it was soaked and dripping.

I lifted my eyes to the mirror, they were dilated and black. Terror filled me as I realized what was happening. The raised area had broken open again. I was horrified.

Blood splashed back on me before I realized it had hit the mirror and countertop. It scattered across my abdomen, shoulder and cheek as if it were a fire hose blasting at short range. I blinked twice, trying to shake myself from the daze I was in.

There was already a large red pool on the floor at my feet. Stepping in it, I slipped, momentarily losing my balance, my arms flailing wildly. I caught myself on the edge of the counter and secured my footing. Then, placing one hand in front of the stream, I quickly moved it inward, trying to control the flow. Instead, blood spattered back at me, adding to my already blood-covered body. I was beginning to look like a character from a horror film.

With my hand firmly over the lesion, I reached for a towel on the shelf behind me, blood dripping from underneath my hand. Anxiously, I pressed it to my chest, freeing up my blood-covered hand so I could try and wash it off in the sink.

I called for Mike. He did not stir. I hesitated doing it again because I did not want to frighten him out of a deep sleep, but I was terrified. I grabbed another, smaller towel and doused it with water and began wiping up the blood. It was all over—on the mirror, in the seam between the sink and countertop, spattered across the faucet and down the front of the cabinet. Then there was the floor; it was smeared all over with footprints detailing every step I had taken.

It hit me oddly that I was cleaning. My only thought was that it could be difficult for Mike to wake up and walk in on the mess. I did not want to see that reaction, so I kept wiping. I had already saturated a hand towel and two washcloths. I called out for him again, my panic increasing. I heard nothing from the other room so I repeated my pleading.

"Mike! I need you!" I yelled a bit louder.

The blood was not slowing. I could feel my skin growing warm underneath the towel as I wiped and wiped, and my heart began to pound harder with the effort. Suddenly, I was exhausted. It was more than the fact that I had just awakened from a deep sleep; it was more than the feelings of an already fatigued body ... it was something else that I could not quite understand, but I kept wiping anyway—my towel now a bright scarlet red.

I pulled the towel away from my chest; the blood was still spewing from the laceration. I quickly pressed another, clean towel to the lesion. Throwing the soiled towel in the hamper, I kept wiping—the front of the cabinets, the mirror again, the counter top. Near where it met the wall, it smeared, but it was the best I could do with one hand.

I wiped the mirror a third time. It streaked a wipe pattern on the glass. I was beginning to feel very nervous as my body temperature continued to rise, and beads of perspiration began dripping from my face. It never even occurred to me that my movements were intensifying the issue.

"Mike!" I said a little louder as I grabbed the edge of the counter and stopped to breathe. "Mike. I need you. Get up." I was feeling weaker.

I heard the crackle of the down comforter and knew he was beginning to stir.

I called to him again, louder still. "Mike, get up! I need you. Can you wake up?" I tried not to sound as hysterical as I was beginning to feel. The bleeding was not slowing.

The mattress squeaked. It was a familiar sound and I knew Mike was getting out of bed. I heard his feet hit the floor and then the door burst open.

"What? What's wrong?" he asked in a nervous voice as he squinted, trying to let his eyes adjust to the overhead light he had just flipped on.

"I'm bleeding again!" I said much less calmly than I wanted to. I pulled the towel away and laid it on the counter as I leaned as far over the sink as I could. He easily saw how saturated it had become and that blood was gushing from my body. I did not mention the other towel I had already discarded or the blood I had wiped up.

I leaned into the sink a little further, shocked that the blood was still draining so profusely. Mike could tell I was scared. I decided he looked alarmed too. It must have been an overwhelming sight. I had blood all over my hands, there was still some marbled across the floor where I had tried to wipe it, and more still on the mirror and cabinets.

He stood there staring, bleary-eyed and said in a slightly elevated tone. "What can I do?"

"Get me a washcloth please," I said, pointing to the shelf.

He grabbed a big yellow towel instead and handed it to me, seemingly unaware of what I had requested. I did not care, I just took it and rolled it up and put it against the edge of the counter so I could lean on it; the stone countertop was cold to the touch.

"Is it old blood again? It looks like old blood," he said, answering his own question.

The thought seemed logical. I reasoned that it was just more collected blood from a leaky capillary.

"Maybe if you let it bleed for a few minutes, it will stop like last time," he suggested, moving closer and holding my shoulders in an effort to steady me.

I thought he might be right and responded, "Maybe you're right," I said hopefully.

He stood there, not moving for a moment or two, then stooped to collect the towels I had dropped on the floor and the one I had thrown in the hamper. He turned and walked back into the bedroom. I heard the laundry room door open and the knob on the washer being twisted around in preparation of starting a new load. Then I heard the water come on.

My back was starting to hurt since I had been leaning over the sink at an awkward angle, so I adjusted myself. I looked at my reflection. There was still blood on my face. I reached up with my free hand and tried to wipe it off, but it was dry and did not budge. It was like watching a motion picture—a bit removed from reality. I stared as the blood drained from my body, and then I began to feel separated from reality.

Everything started to whirl and spin. Looking down at my chest it dawned on me; the blood was not old, it was new ... and my body was still using it! I began to feel faint and I knew if I did not get to the floor immediately, I was going to blackout and fall. Then, without the ability to put pressure on the open sore, I would bleed to death right here on my own bathroom floor.

Grabbing the edge of the countertop to steady my wobbly knees, I moved swiftly, relocating myself, down onto the cold tile, nearly losing consciousness. I managed to grab a towel on my way down and pressed it to my chest. Then I rolled to my back.

I had heard about people seeing stars before. I never had … until now. They were sparking and dancing in an eddy of misty white that rotated over my head. I felt dizzy and my body felt numb and vacant; in fact, it felt like I was dying.

I had never really considered what dying might feel like. As it brushed up against me now, I thought how strangely calm it was. All of a sudden, everything seemed far away. Colors became muted and sounds were only echoes to my ears. I tried to call Mike's name, but nothing came out. I felt my mouth moving, yet there was no sound. The bathroom light shone down from the ceiling, glistening through a sea of stars. I listened internally as my heart beat a rhythmic pattern, steadily slowing. It was the only clear sound I could perceive. I breathed in and attempted to call for Mike again.

A whisper slipped past my lips. "Mike," I said weakly, knowing he would not hear me. I breathed in; it seemed slow and labored, but I tried again. "Mike." It came out a little louder this time as I concentrated on putting more air behind it.

Seconds later, he was standing at my side. I reached a hand toward him. He took it looking as though he could see me slipping away. All I could say was "Help me." It seemed an involuntary comment, and almost like someone else had said it. Then I closed my eyes.

"Alicia!" His voice rang in my ears. "What do I do?"

I felt him rolling me carefully to one side and slipping a towel underneath my body, creating a barrier between the frigid tile and me. He placed another under my head for a pillow, and then another over my shivering, half-naked body.

I heard the window shut just above me and knew he had closed it to keep the cold night air from blowing in on me.

I internally questioned how cold it was. It was winter in the mountains of Utah after all.

Mike kneeled down next to me, "Should I take you to the hospital?" he asked, his voice sounding tense.

Just as I was considering his question, I began to feel a little better, and I said, "No. I think I'll be okay, just give me a minute." Things began to clear and my senses were returning. Then, slowly, a feeling of peace came over me and I knew everything was going to be all right.

Mike was uncertain of my declaration. He had shifted to his knees and was holding my hand. I could tell by his voice that he was ready to jump if I said the word.

"Let me just lay here for a few minutes. I think I'll be okay; I'm feeling a lot better. Go lay down, I'll call if I need you," I said in my normal voice. The frailty I had been experiencing seemed to diminish quickly.

He hesitated, answering me, "Are ... are you sure?"

My eyes were still closed, but I nodded, expecting that he would see it.

"Okay," his voice sounded uncertain and tentative, but he started getting up anyway. "I'm going to lie down on the foot of the bed; it's only ten feet away. Call me if you need anything," he said as he stood and walked out of the room. I heard the mattress squeak.

I am certain he questioned leaving the room, but I also knew he was not fully awake. I was glad he took my encouragement to lay down. I knew he was not a good sleeper and I worried about him, even in this strange circumstance.

After a while, I began to feel strength returning to my body. I realized that lying down had taken the pressure off the open wound, allowing it to coagulate. As soon as I felt better, maybe ten or fifteen minutes later, I was ready to move back to the bed.

"Mike?" I called. "Can you come and help me get up?"

A few seconds later he was next to me. "Here, let me help you," he said, supporting the arm I had already planted onto the tile floor in an attempt to push myself up.

"Thank you," I said.

He put one hand behind my back, lifting me to a sitting position. Then, when I indicated I was all right, he helped me to my feet. He grabbed a fresh towel and laid it to my chest so I could take it with me—just in case. Gently he laid me down on the mattress and covered me with the quilt. I quickly fell asleep.

~

The next morning when I awoke, I felt okay—surprisingly. But I had not tried to get out of bed yet. I expected to be weak or lightheaded, at the very least. Mike heard me rouse and rolled over, looking at me.

"How do you feel?" he asked as he touched my arm. I wondered if he had gotten any sleep at all; he looked tired.

"Better, I think," I replied, wondering.

"I'm glad to hear that. You had me pretty scared last night," he said.

"I had me pretty scared last night," I retorted with a weak grin.

"Maybe you should text Don today. I bet he'd have some idea what that was all about."

I nodded, then thought about his suggestion, deliberating about it for quite a while. It still worried me to disturb Don at home and I wondered what I would say, knowing full well that I was not paying him for his time. I began rehearsing what I would text to him. "Hey Don, I almost passed out and bled to death last night." No, that sounded trite and flippant, not to mention it was a little too descriptive. I thought about just saying, "I lost a lot of blood last night," but talked myself out of it since it did not seem descriptive enough. Then it occurred to me to keep it simple, pique his curiosity, and then pray that he might want to call me. That way it was not laying any of my emotional pressure on him.

I typed out the comment, "I had a scary experience last night," then hit the send button. The next thing I knew, my phone was ringing.

Don asked what was going on, and after I had detailed the entire ordeal, he reiterated that the blood was indeed coming from a broken capillary. He had seen it before. That made me feel a lot better, and then he gave me some ideas on how to replenish my body's red blood cells quickly so I could regain my strength.

He said, "You'll need to either drink some coconut water, or you can mix two raw, organic cage-free eggs with organic grape juice and drink that. That's what they do in other countries instead of giving transfusions."

I had never heard of such a concoction before, but was open to trying anything. I thanked him profusely, and immediately sent Mike to the store.

Throughout the rest of the day, I researched what had happened to me. From everything I read, and my near fainting physical response to the blood loss, it likely amounted to about two quarts. That was nearly half of all the blood in my entire body. I wondered what another ten minutes of losing more blood would have done. The thought made me shudder.

Chapter Twenty-One

WHEN YOU LEAST EXPECT IT

The day after my scary experience, I stopped taking the pain medication. I managed, but going without certainly did not stop the pain. As per Don's instructions, I drank large quantities of raw tart cherry juice and sucked on frozen cherries in an effort to alleviate the relentless ache. I believed fully that the pain would subside as the medication left my system. What I did not realize was that my body had become rather accustomed to what I had been giving it. Determination or not, it turned out to be much more difficult than anticipated.

Something Don had said stuck with me, "It's hard to heal." I took those words to mean more than just physical healing. Through this journey, everything in me was healing—my mind, body, and spirit. Even though I could feel myself changing, Satan was right there in times of weakness, infusing negative expressions, causing me to vacillate again.

The voices were loud, "Your faith is not strong enough!" and "You'll never be able to reach your desired goal; you might as well give up and go see a doctor." They hit me right where it hurt, in my weakest place—my faith. "It takes a much better person than you to accomplish such a feat of spiritual strength. That is reserved for people more important than you."

As the words stung my consciousness, I thought of spiritual leaders like Mother Teresa and Gandhi, whom I expected were more faith-filled than I; thus, the voices were somewhat effective in discouraging me. When I finally recognized that the words were not Godly in nature, I, again, took steps to alter my thinking by pushing back as hard as I could. It constantly amazed me how easy it was for darkness to creep in—and so quickly.

Two days after the blood loss, my determination for complete pill freedom was seriously waning. Mike came in at his usual time that evening and found me on the bed in the spare room curled up into a tight ball, crying and writhing in torment.

"Honey," he said. His voice sounded despondent. He sat carefully on the edge of the bed so he would not cause any shaking, and lifted my head gently, cradling me in his arms. "You can't do this! It's too much to ask. Please take some medication," he begged.

My first thought was of Don. It terrified me that he might not work with me if I could not quit the medication. I thought about Mike's offer for all of three seconds and mumbled, "Okay."

My heart swelled with both grief and joy; it killed me that I was failing to accomplish the task at hand, and yet I was joyful knowing I would feel better soon.

"You can cut the pills back gradually," Mike offered.

I realized as he said it, that the pain I was feeling was not from the tumor, it was not exclusive to my chest area as it had been before. This was much more intense and included my entire body; my legs hurt, my toes hurt, my skin hurt, even my hair hurt. And then it dawned on me—I was going through chemical dependence withdrawal.

I had been on so many pills that my body had learned to rely on them. It made me angry with myself. All I needed was one more thing to complicate my life. I wanted to tell Mike what I had just realized, but my energy was tapped out and I could not hold a conversation.

He carefully laid me back on the bed and left the room. Moments later he returned with three pills—a big step down from my previous dose—and a glass of water. Gratefully I took them. He covered me with the blanket, kissed me, and left me to rest. It took at least an hour for the pain to begin relenting, and then I fell asleep.

Two hours later I awoke. I felt somewhat improved. Mike heard me and stepped in from the kitchen. "Hey, how are you feeling?" he asked softly as he sat down on the foot of the bed.

I took in a breath. "Better; beat up though," I replied quietly. Then I took another breath and weakly said, "I figured out what was going on—that was withdrawal." I felt exhausted from the short conversation and closed my eyes.

"I know," he said, moving closer to me. "That was my thought, too. Something was different this time."

I opened my eyes and looked at him, nodding feebly.

By the look on his face, I could see he was hurting with me.

"I feel bad for you," he said, leaning in carefully and kissing my cheek, "I'm glad you're feeling better. I guess you know you have to reduce your pills slowly and spread it out over time, right?" He looked tentative, like he thought I would be upset by his judiciously worded question.

I nodded again and said, "Don told me that healing is uncomfortable. He was right."

Mike offered to fix me a plate of food. I was surprised how hungry I was and agreed.

He smiled and stood gently, then walked out the door.

After a few days, I figured out how to reduce my pills sensibly. I noticed that as I took the dosage down, the pain seemed to come down with it. I decided Don was right about pills causing pain. I did not completely quit at that time, but felt a lot better about the number I was now taking and vowed that I would eventually get rid of them all.

~

By mid-January, the raised area on my breast had turned into an all-out eruption. There was no more blood loss, thank goodness, but just like a demonic possession, the top layer of skin had broken wide open and the tumor was literally emerging, rising from the depths of its core and exorcizing itself right there onto my chest. In some ways it encouraged me, but in others, it terrified me; the images of those disfigured women from so many months before seeped in. With or without chemo and radiation, I knew *this* could permanently disfigure me.

I kept a record of the progress of the tumor as it arose. It stunned me when I took measurements; it protruded a full inch, was one-and-a-half inches from left to right, and another three inches from top to bottom.

Dr. Howard's comment about the tumor being the size of an orange echoed in my ears. It was a small orange, but it was still an orange. I could see it, not just in my mind's eyes, but literally. The uncertainty caused my faith to swing radically. I was sapped by the emotional roller coaster that had plagued me since the beginning of the year. I was tired and wanted to quit, but could not. I still had knowledge that I would heal, but the unknowns pounded with unyielding repetition. Physically and mentally I was taxed to the point of numbness, and I worried frequently that I would not be strong enough. It was another massive exposure of my perceived weak faith.

Several times a day I was hit with a forced self-examination of whether or not I had the mettle to trust God. I was the only one who had the ability to give up fear for faith, and even though I had *knowledge* of the eventual outcome, it was still a battle when the pain blew in.

Strangely, and despite everything, there was a pervasive sense of tranquility. I found myself confused by the diametrically opposed sensations. It was as though my spirit and my body were in constant conflict; my spirit wanting me to heal and giving me the sense of the spiritual, and my body refusing to bend to the suggestion.

As would happen sometimes, I would find myself cornered by the sadness of it all. One evening Mike was in the kitchen making something to eat as I had just shuffled across the room and into the living area. The television was humming. Nothing in particular was happening, but all of a sudden, without any provocation, I was hit with a wave of grief that crippled me.

Swelling from somewhere deep within my soul, it came. If I could give it a color it would have been sharp neon blue, like the flame of a fire. It heated up, worked its way up my throat, and boiled into the air around me; it left me gasping for air.

By the time I comprehended what was happening, it was too late to intervene. My entire body was involved and unexpectedly overcome by a crushing sadness that drew itself around me so quickly that there was no chance of escape.

I heaved in and grabbed the back of the couch with one hand, barely able to catch a breath, and my eyes instantly filled with liquid that burned as it brimmed and fell down my cheeks. It was as if someone had popped a cork on every emotion that had piled up during the preceding few weeks. A peculiar voice broke into the room, blistering my ears with its shrill and pain-filled sounds. Mike's chin shot up and his eyes locked on me, a look of shock spreading across his face.

I drew in another huge breath, placed both hands on the back of the couch so as not to fall, and spewed out sounds that shot forth from me like an explosion of fireworks.

I reached up, covering my mouth with both hands, and doubled over at the waist, trying to stop the mounting pain. I had not heard myself wrench in this kind of demonstrative agony for a long, long time. In fact, I could count on one hand the times in my life where noises from my very depths assaulted my ears as these did. It was as though the dark one himself had put his hand right down my throat, dragged the sounds out, and threw them down at my feet. I could almost see him stepping back callously and laughing.

My knees started to fold and my skull throbbed; I felt myself falling. In an instant Mike was at my side, as soon as it registered what was happening. He grabbed me just as my knees were completely giving out and pulled me into his body for support; my arms curled across my chest as I hung there like a rag doll. Mike never let go. He just held me squarely in his grasp.

I have no recollection of how long I hung there crying, but it was a while. As my senses slowly returned and I was able to put my feet under me, I could feel Mike's breath warm against my neck; it was soothing. The fact that he was simply there absorbing my pain created a bond between us that will last far beyond any earth life. He had told me he would be there no matter what but, until now, I had not truly believed it—not completely. But here he was, literally buoying me up and silently sharing every shard of pain I was experiencing. I had never treasured him more at any point in our lives.

I heaved, broken cries scattering the quiet as we sat down on the couch.

He softly whispered, "I can't say that I didn't see it coming." Moments later another wave moved in, bringing another gush of sobs and tears that racked my body in unrestrained convulsions. Mike tightened his hold and said, "I'm here."

The pain loosened its clutch on me and moved slowly away from my heart, and all the while Mike just kept hugging me.

After what seemed like forever, I finally calmed and began breathing normally again. My limbs were weak and exhausted. I never moved though. I lingered in Mike's arms, attempting to be cleansed and filled with his love. I basked in the warmth he emanated, selfishly taking what I needed. He never budged. He never faltered. He just held me there until I was strong enough.

Chapter Twenty-Two

PHOTOGRAPHING THE EVIDENCE

Aside from a few business trips during the previous year, I had steady and constant attendance at church. I knew it would only be a matter of time before someone realized I was not just out of town. A few weeks into my absence, that is exactly what happened.

Mike came home from church to report that this person or that had asked of my whereabouts. He dutifully explained that I was ill. I could see in his eyes the yearning to tell them more so that he might not carry the burden alone. That weighed heavily on me. It had to be hard for him to hold the information so close, but I was unwilling to open that door just yet.

He moved into the kitchen and laid his keys on the counter.

"The bishop asked me if we'd found any health insurance yet," Mike started. "I told him how difficult it had been to find anything affordable, and he said I should keep looking."

With that little bit of continued encouragement, Mike set out on an Internet-driven quest to find insurance for me. He believed the dually mentioned counsel from the bishop to be spiritual direction. So, for the next two weeks, he spent hours online searching.

One night he announced, "I found some insurance for you and they'll back date it to the first of the year."

It was almost in passing so I did not really pay attention. The only thought I had was it would be an unnecessary expense on our already tight budget.

Plus, I had not been to the doctor at all that year, so the backdating did not matter to me. Oddly, I did not intend to go to a doctor either. The act of putting insurance in place slammed up against my denial of all the possibilities.

Somehow, though, I felt a strange sense of relief. The word "procedure" popped in again, too. I chose not to acknowledge its presence. That would be like admitting I was going to need the insurance. Unbeknown to me, the Lord had always known what I would need. In big ways and small, He just kept answering my prayers—even if I failed to recognize or accept some of them.

~

As my body continued to morph, I resorted to dressing in Mike's button-up shirts with a varied selection of black yoga pants. I had dropped more weight, so the pants I was used to putting on were too big, and my own shirts were completely out of the question as they had become too confining and uncomfortable.

I made my way to the couch and glanced out the window to the north. The stark beauty of winter had mostly been swallowed up in the grayness of my circumstances. I had missed much of it. It had turned icy and cold and the sun streaked in between the clouds, bringing a subconscious hint of new life and spring. Pulling a blanket over my lap, I heard a tiny knock on the door, and then it opened.

Jill, my daughter, bounced in, all bubbles and smiling. "Hi, Mum," she said with that cute annotation on the "um" part she always used. Her arms were loaded with multiple bags so she kicked the front door closed with her foot. Shuffling to the kitchen, she began unloading groceries. It felt good to have her nearby.

My phone buzzed. It was Don. We had been communicating via text all that morning. When his schedule opened up a while after that, he called. I told him how the raised area was growing daily, and how disturbed I was by its appearance. When I finished he said, "I don't mean to be offensive, but could you send me a picture of it?"

I choked a bit. It set me back that he would want to see it, but I was in no way offended. It smacked me hard as I comprehended that he had no idea what I was really dealing with. I had never detailed it for him. I only called it the "raised area." I swallowed hard.

Looking at Jill with wide eyes, I saw her reaction. It was one of surprise, but then she nodded ever so slightly. My phone was on speaker mode so she heard Don's question.

"Sure, I guess so. It's pretty gross," I said to Don, wondering if he would be sickened by the appearance of what was happening on my chest.

"I'll call you afterward," he said. I heard the phone disconnect.

I turned to Jill, knowing that she was going to have to help me take the photo. "Oh, wow. You ready for this?" I asked, worrying about how seeing it might affect her.

Her face contorted slightly and she forced a smirk, "Actually, I have a morbid curiosity about it. So, yes," she said.

When I revealed to her what I had been dealing with, all she could say was, "Wow." I could not blame her. There really were no words to describe it.

The photo was carefully taken so that my modesty would still be intact. A few minutes after sending the images to Don from my smart phone, he sent four photographs back to me of other people who had horrific growths that looked just like mine—either on their neck or chin. They looked exactly like what I was dealing with, except theirs were much, much larger. That gave me *great* courage.

Don called about two minutes later. As I picked up the phone, I found myself nervously fumbling with it before I could even answer. When I finally did, Don said, "I didn't know it was that bad." My heart sank. I imagined him telling me that there was no hope and that it was too far gone, and that it was beyond anything he'd ever seen, but that is not what happened.

"Obviously, I've seen this before—many, many times," he began. My emotions swung wildly again, this time to the side of confidence. His voice was strong and sure, and it did not have the slightest waver. And then he said, "You're going to be just fine."

Tears flooded my eyes and words stammered through me. "Wait, what? What did you just say? I'm going to be fine?" I almost asked him to say it again. I drew in lungs full of air and bit my lip and smiled at Jill. Tears dripped down my face.

That one small comment pushed away every shard of terror that remained in my heart, and I was filled with peace. Even though I knew the Lord had already told me I would be fine, hearing the words from someone who had seen what I was dealing with before caused my entire body to electrify. I wanted to jump for joy! God was answering my fears through Don, and the sound in his voice soothed me as if Jesus Christ himself was delivering the message to me.

I sat stunned, holding in the sounds that were gurgling just behind my voice box. Jill looked at me and smiled too. We listened to Don tell a story about one of the photos.

The photo reflected a tumor the size of a cauliflower attached to the right side of a woman's neck. It was so large that she could hardly hold her own head up. In a second picture, there was a tall, slender blonde woman with pretty blue eyes and a warm smile. She was standing next to Don, who had his arm around her.

"Those two photos are of the same woman," Don declared. I looked at Jill and then darted from one photo to the other trying to see the comparison. "She was told by her doctors that she was going to die within two months, but that they could expand it to four if she consented to chemotherapy and radiation. She and her husband had two small children at the time and her husband begged her to do it. He didn't want her to die yet. He said that a few more months were better than nothing."

"She told him that she'd heard I was coming to town and wanted to come to one of my events. If after attending, there was still no chance, she would take the doctor's advice and begin chemotherapy."

Jill looked at me, her eyes wide with interest.

Don continued, "Well, she came to my event and afterward we talked. I gave her some protocols to follow and she went home and followed them. I hadn't heard from her again until I happened to be in that city again for another event. As soon as I stepped on stage, she came running up, took the microphone right out of my hands, and proceeded to tell everyone what I had taught her and how it had saved her life."

"Whoa," I said wiping my face, "that's incredible."

"It's not that incredible," Don said. "People just don't know what to do because they've been so brainwashed into thinking there isn't another way. So they turn their lives over to someone they hope and pray knows what to do. And, often, they don't. They're just *practicing*." He accentuated the last word with a goofy, cartoon sounding voice. It resonated in my ears.

Don continued talking, "If you don't mind, I want to send your photo to a few oncologist friends of mine so we can discuss what you're dealing with."

Initially I was surprised at his request, wondering why he would have anything to do with the medical profession at all. Then he explained, "These particular doctors left their professional careers after coming to my lectures. They learned that they could save more lives with whole-food healing and holistic approaches."

My mouth just hung open. I was shocked and impressed and completely taken aback by the idea of someone actually leaving something they had worked so long for. It gave me immediate and deep respect for those men who chose to quit, based on truth and not the money.

"I want to get their recommendations, if that's all right with you," he said.

I nodded, as though he could see me over the phone, and then I remembered to breathe. "Yes. I would like to know what they say," concluding that it would be very valuable to have both sides of the spectrum covered—the natural and the medical.

As the call came to an end, Don made some recommendations as to what I could do immediately and told me he'd get back to me in less than a week. That very afternoon I began a protocol of applying tea tree oil topically on the wound and surrounding skin, as per his suggestions. Four days passed and I noticed that my healthy skin was starting to react. The skin was peeling again, but below the growth in a different area. My imagination began running wild and I visualized the tumor emerging from that other place. I grabbed my phone and quickly shot a text off to Don. I had to wait for a few hours before he responded, during which time, I was ticking off all the possibilities. To say they freaked me out would be an understatement.

When he called, he gave me a few more ideas, which I was eager to try. I trusted Don. His ideas and suggestions were all practical solutions to physical issues that had actually worked for people he knew. And the confidence in his voice encouraged me on. I prayed often, thanking the Lord for Don's entrance into my life. I felt like I had been given a treasure of great knowledge. I instantly appreciated the years of study it took for Don to uncover all that he now knew. I felt in my heart that when—*not if*—I got through this, Heavenly Father would use me to help others acquire and understand the power of what I was now learning.

~

Physically, things were getting harder for me. Although I had spiritual confidence and a growing knowledge that was firmly in place, I still had to deal with my shifting condition from day to day. It felt like I had stopped living and only existed. My world grew smaller and only revolved around my physical needs. I felt like I was living in a box. It was disheartening.

Just as I had felt the previous December, I knew *it* was coming—something more. It loomed in my brain, far enough out of reach that I could not really grasp a timeframe. And even though I constantly reminded myself that this situation would only be a small moment in the overall scheme of my life, it did not help the fear I felt, knowing I was closer as the days wore on.

Mom called quite a lot around that time, which certainly helped to break up the monotony of the days. We had always been close and I knew that she intuitively sensed that I was struggling. For whatever reason, I became closed again and worked to keep most of my feelings from her. Her calls became more frequent, occurring several times a day. Sometimes it would chafe me because I did not want to tell her how I was, but I was certain she already knew.

One morning she asked if I needed her to come down. That was exactly what I wanted, but I heard myself say, "No. I'll be okay." I'm not sure why I was so unwilling to invite and welcome her. I guess I kept thinking that everything was about to turn in the other direction. In my stubborn independence, I thought I could do it alone.

Dad called two days later. The second I heard his voice, I knew that Mom had put him up to it. Her instincts were always correct. Mom knew that ever since I was a child, Dad knew how to get into my heart. He did it that day, too.

"Wouldn't you like your mother there?" he asked.

"I'm doing okay, Dad," I lied, trying to hide my feelings.

"Well, she'd really like to come help you anyway," he responded, easily detecting the slight shades of grey in my response. "I'll bet you could use a little help, couldn't you?" he asked, poking holes in my stubbornness.

"Well …," I started, and then I stopped mid-sentence, wondering if I should really expose my real situation. Before I had a chance to put together a cohesive thought, he said, "We could be there in a few days, if you'll let me bring her."

His offer touched a nerve as a strange relief flooded over me. It took all I had to remain composed. Inside I yelled, "If I'll let you? Yes! Yes, I'll let you. I need her! Please bring her down." But instead, I said, "Okay."

Dad knew exactly how to get to me. Three days later, they were on my doorstep.

That was a hard day for me. I was in bed, twisting in pain. I texted the code to the front door so I would not have to get out of bed to let them in. When they walked into the bedroom where I was lying, they appeared shocked.

Their reactions set me back, drawing the fear out of my heart again. It swelled, gripping me in a rush of darkness. Distress quickly spread across my face. I watched them take note and quickly shove their emotions somewhere I could not see.

Mom dropped everything and began organizing everything, including making a list of my needs. Dad went outside, carrying in a few things from the car. One item was a beanbag covered in green and gold paisley fabric. He heated it in the microwave for a few minutes and then delivered it to me, announcing that it was a last minute item he grabbed, thinking it might help.

As I pressed the bag to my chest, it began absorbing the heat. Relief radiated into my entire body and suddenly I could breathe again. My lungs expanded fully, cleansing and bringing the reprieve I was in such desperate need of. I exhaled loudly. It was fresh and replenishing, and then there was no pain . . . none. My whole body sighed with relief.

"It's helping!" I said, a tear trickling down my cheek.

I said a silent prayer of thankfulness. I knew that the Lord had prompted him to bring it. It took me only seconds to see that those who loved and cared for me were my living angels.

~

A few days later, before he left to go home, Dad stepped into the bedroom where I was curled up with a blanket. I was in a lot of pain, wincing at any movement I made.

He stepped carefully to my side, trying hard not to touch the mattress or jar it in any way. He stood there for a time just staring at me, in that small space between the bed and the wall, then he leaned in, gently placing his hands on my face. For a long time, he just held me, softly rubbing my cheeks. I was sure I sensed a level of pain from him. I could only imagine what he was thinking; his only daughter, lying there on what, I expect, looked like death's door. His hands felt good and were a welcome distraction from my former pain-focused attention.

"Can I give you a blessing?" he asked as he took his hands from my face.

I moaned a reply, "Yes."

Dad laid his hands on my head. He mentioned healing and diminishment of the pain, and an increase in my effort to rely on Heavenly Father.

When finished, he removed his hands and leaned in, kissing my cheek. "I love you," he said. Then he brushed the hair to the side of my face and smiled.

"I love you too, Dad," I said.

Over the next two hours, after Dad had left, the pain declined. A little in awe of the hand of God in the moment, I secretly prayed—for a long, long time—thanking God for the relief. It was another powerful manifestation of how real the powers of heaven could be in my life. I was learning to trust the Lord more completely during my suffering. Somehow, I think that was the point of it all.

Chapter Twenty-Three

SALT OF THE EARTH

Since *not* dying was my goal, I governed my life as if I were in a long-distance marathon, focusing on the task in front of me. When I reached a goal, I would set my sights further ahead and move on to next one. It had become difficult, but I was resolute.

The directive to move my body daily, which Don had given me, seemed unreachable. Although there were times when I found solace in my situation, there was a larger portion that was simply pain-filled, so when Don had said, "Movement is life. You have to move. I want you to walk outside every day," I was pretty sure it would kill me.

Slowly shifting my own body weight from side to side was a chore. I analyzed what he said for a few minutes and then realized the converse of what he was telling me—non-movement meant death. That was the opposite of my objective, so like an obstinate child unwilling to pick up her toys, I hunkered down, crossed my arms, and refused the choice of death.

Movement equated to a lot pain. Every step I took, every budge, every movement vibrated in me like a million spears piercing my skin from the inside out.

Don repeatedly said, "It doesn't matter if you can only walk for a few minutes, you have to do it, and then you can build up from there."

Mike began taking me out after work to walk but, I confess, I did not want to go. It was excruciating and I was weak and bent. But I knew I had to.

Every evening Mom or Mike would slowly pry me from off the couch and help me hobble to a nearby chair. I would sit near the edge as Mom slipped a snow boot on one foot while Mike pushed on the other. Then Mom would rush to the microwave and heat the beanbag so that I could shove it inside my coat to help keep me warm and, hopefully, help lessen the pain.

Mom had brought a size "medium" coat with her, but she did not know why. She knew I had plenty of coats, and knew I was nowhere near a medium anymore. Even before I began to lose weight, it would have been big on me, but now it completely swamped me. It quickly became apparent that it was another blessing from God. Although my body was wasting away, the tumor had grown large enough that the extra space of the larger coat made it closable. My own coats would not have accommodated the extra bulk, plus the beanbag.

That first time outside in over a month, Mike helped me cross the threshold. As we stepped into the night air, I breathed as deeply as my lungs could handle. I could not remember the last time cold penetrated me like that. The air burned my eyes and the skin on my face awakened. Reminding me what it felt like to feel something other than physical pain.

The frozen sidewalks crunched beneath my boots. My legs were tenuous and shaky but Mike held me tightly, as though I were a ninety-year-old woman crossing a busy intersection. I glanced up at him; steam was rising from his mouth as he focused on the roadway in front of us.

"Thank you for him. He is my rock. I love him so much more than I can say," I prayed.

I stumbled slightly and moaned at the quiver it caused. Mike's grip tightened on my arm and he slowed a little. I took another step, the shuffling motion rattling me. I gasped and then whimpered again. Mike stopped. He looked down and said, "Are you all right?"

I wanted to scream that I wasn't all right, but I did not. I just nodded in the affirmative.

We did not move for a minute, waiting for me to catch my breath. One of my arms was interlocked with his, and the other was pressed heavily against my chest, trying to moderate each tremor. There was no question about it—walking hurt.

Don's voice rang in my ears. He had said, "It's uncomfortable to heal."

That brought me comfort. It did not take a day to get where I was, so I was going to have to suffer the costs of my sick body and allow the time and discomfort it was going to take to heal. I was to do everything I could to help myself, if I expected the Lord to heal me.

I breathed deeply again and noticed the glorious scent of balsam from a burning fireplace somewhere. The moon was full and cast a silvery glow on the snow. There was a jagged streak of smoke strewn across the cloudless sky. Every nerve in my body was electrified, and began coming to life, invigorating my spirit enough that I was actually eager to continue. It felt good to be outside of my little world. And even though it was not a leisurely stroll on the walking path that weaved itself throughout our neighborhood, I found that I was happy to be there. We probably only walked thirty or forty yards but I did it. It was a small triumph and I felt recharged.

"I can do this," I said out loud as we muddled our way back home.

"Yes, you can," Mike added.

A small smile spread across my face and a fire reignited inside of me. For the first time in a long time I felt positive and mentally stronger; I knew I could do whatever it was going to take.

As we stepped back into the house, I kept repeating Don's comment to myself like a chant, "It's uncomfortable to heal; it's uncomfortable to heal. It's uncomfortable to heal."

That gave me a shift in thinking. Because I knew that I was going to be uncomfortable, I could see the difficult journey ahead; however, I *was* going to heal.

~

I had been applying raw honey directly to the open wound, per Don's instructions. I was not certain what it was supposed to do, but the expectation was that it would help somehow. A week into the applications, I told Don there was no noticeable change.

His response was, "I wish you could do salt packs," as if I knew what he meant.

My brow rutted and my mouth twisted sideways. I was confused. "What are salt packs?"

He proceeded to explain that it meant applying a generous amount of salt directly to the wound. He was very specific as to the kind of salt I should use, "Not just any salt, but *good* sea salt," he stated. "I've seen it work miracles!"

I was encouraged by his testament and had Mike pick some up on his way home from work. I packed the tumor with salt that very night.

The very next morning, my heart about leaped into my throat, nearly gagging me as I gulped in a spluttered breath and shouted my findings. "Mom, come here!" I screamed.

I heard her footsteps hit the floor near the couch as she hastened toward me. She stopped short of the bathroom door, which was closed, then asked, "What is it? Are you okay?"

I could feel her tension right through the door. Not wanting to leave her hanging, I said, "You aren't going to believe this, but the tumor is changing!" I said loudly.

Peeling back the covering, I found something was very different; the top layer of the tumor looked as though it were developing a scab. It had darkened and dried, and looked like an old pair of leather shoes that had been left in the sun for too long.

"What?" she asked with a high-pitched twang, "In a good or a bad way?"

"Good, I think," I responded. Then I began describing what I was seeing.

"Finally," I said. "Maybe this is the top of the mountain and I can start going down now."

In an instant, I could finally see the end of the tunnel.

Over the course of the next few days, things changed dramatically. The tumor began to emerge at a quicker rate than ever before. The pain increased, but my faith was firmly set and I could see visible changes daily. Irrespective of the discomfort, I was encouraged.

Chapter Twenty-Four

YELLING AT GOD

I was still taking a few pain pills. I had also added white willow bark capsules, hoping that a more natural pain reliever would diminish my suffering.

One particular afternoon, the pain bashed me like a tidal wave pounding the surf, never ending and growing in intensity until it practically dashed me into unconsciousness. As it rose in my body, I began to entertain some very dark ideas about death as an escape. No doubt it was Satan taking advantage of the fact that I was so besieged by pain.

Sitting there on the couch, I hugged my knees tight to my chest until there was little room to breathe. Slowly, I rocked myself back and forth, moaning from the very depths of the hell I was in. There was no escape. I accepted the pain like a long thorn that could not be removed.

I heard my mother stand. She had been seated a few feet away from me on the couch. I did not open my eyes. They remained tightly closed and I remained securely imprisoned.

The next thing I realized, she was standing behind me. Lightly she pressed her hands on each side of my skull. I could hear her breathing heavily, although it sounded far away and distant. I knew she was crying. Small noises slipped from her lips and one of her tears fell onto my cheek. I shuddered, which brought me back into the moment and I began to sense my surroundings again. Mom was in as much agony as I. Instinctively, I knew she was praying.

Although I did not hear her prayer, I did notice something happen rather quickly. Within minutes, there was a lessening in the overall pressure to my body. The lines that had been pulled tight on my face began to relax. Then I began to feel a sense of release as my breathing slowed.

Within the hour, I was substantially better. The pain was not completely gone, but it was lessened. After a time, I became lucid enough to talk.

I sighed and looked over at Mom who was sitting near my outstretched feet at the opposite end of the couch. I could see the weariness on her face. She smiled and said, "That was scary. Are you feeling okay?"

I nodded slightly. "Better," I said. "Hope that never happens again." Then I closed my eyes and attempted to recover a little more.

"I hope not either," Mom said.

I knew I had not reached the peak of this experience and was sure times like these were not over yet. I prayed that the Lord would strengthen my ability to handle what was coming.

I cracked my eyes open and glanced at Mom; she was looking at me compassionately. Mascara was a little smudged under one eye.

She reached over and touched my hand, smiling ever so slightly. Her look was a mixture of pain and relief. I hated seeing her suffer. It made me feel a little guilty for having her come, but I was so very thankful.

"Can I get you anything?" she asked, leaning forward so she could see my face, which was pointed down toward my chest.

"Water?" I responded, licking my parched lips.

She arose from the couch, quickly filling a glass for me.

"I had pretty much had enough of watching you suffer and I couldn't stand it anymore. I had been praying and praying, but it didn't seem to be working. You just kept crying." She choked on the memory and swallowed back a sob. "It was killing me to watch. When I got up and wrapped my hands around your head ..."

She stopped mid-sentence to compose the tears that were brimming at the edge of her eyes. Then she heaved softly a few times. I saw her chin quiver. She reached up and wiped her eyes and cheek as the tears got away. Her anguish penetrated me like a newly sharpened dagger. I forced the sadness downward, stopping its exit from my mouth.

She continued, "When I put my hands around your head, I was still praying." She took a few shallow breaths then. "I was screaming to the Lord. I said, 'Now! We need you now!'"

A single tear rolled down her cheek and I could see a shadow flash across her face as she relived the awfulness of it all. The corners of her mouth were turned down into a slight frown.

Surprising myself, I chuckled lightly and teased, "You yelled at Heavenly Father."

Mom's chin came up and she latched onto my eyes. The solemnity of it all vaporized. Then she chuckled, "Yes, I guess I did." She looked heavenward and said in playful jest, "Sorry."

I smiled through my exhaustion.

"He heard me though," she continued with a relieved smile on her face. "Almost immediately you began to relax."

I nodded. "I know. I could feel that. Guess we chalk it up to the power of a mother's prayer," I responded weakly.

I silently blessed my mother's name and recognized that it was her faith that saved me from an even more horrific experience. The Lord had stepped in and blessed me because of her. I was grateful. Gratitude flooded my spirit, and I nodded off to sleep.

~

It was the first day of February and Mom announced that my brother and his wife were coming down from Idaho to visit. A bizarre and sharp agony shot into my heart like it had taken a blow from a shotgun. My eyes burned and fury awakened within me. "What if they've come to say goodbye because they think I'm going to die?" The words seared onto the front interior of my skull, bringing with it a darkness that enveloped me.

Satan knew me, and he knew exactly which buttons to push in order to re-harness every single fear I had managed to conquer. If he could convince me that someone who loved and cared for me expected my untimely death, it would shatter everything I had come to believe. If he could place even a shred of doubt in me about my healing, he could potentially disrupt my course, and if nothing else, he could watch with humor as I suffered with the internal noise. The weight of the idea grew in me until I was completely incensed.

The more I allowed the negative thoughts to roll around, the more I believed that they were coming to say goodbye. For several hours before their arrival, that thought festered into an ugly, dark cloud that spread over me in varying layers of grey. I could feel the rage building up inside of me until I thought I would pop.

"Why are they coming?" I asked Mom in a tone that caused her to jerk her head up and look at me oddly. "Do they think I'm going to die or something? They never come here." There was unmistakable venom in my voice.

She looked utterly and completely shocked by my line of thinking. Her mouth dropped into an open position as if she were going to say something. She blinked, looked down, took in another breath and then closed her mouth tightly. I could see her thinking, trying to find a way to manage what I had just thrown up all over her.

She drew in a breath and softly explained, "No, they're coming because you're sick and they love you."

If there had been a water balloon above me, it would have burst, saturating me in my own ridiculous comments. Every concern or fear, or misplaced thought was immediately washed away with the imaginary baptism. It left the air around me clean and clear, as though Satan had been washed out with it.

Instantly I could see what was happening. The pendulum had been shoved again in the opposite direction of my confidence. Clarity filled me, and I quickly shoved it back, pushing any and all negative feelings out. I muttered a silent prayer of gratitude, and prayed for forgiveness.

"I'm sorry Mom," I whispered, tears streaking down my face. "I don't believe what I said."

She moved close to me and pulled me to her shoulder. "It's okay, honey. I know you don't really think that way. It was just a weak moment."

I felt ridiculous and embarrassed for my words, but I was so very thankful they happened before my brother came. I heaved in and let my tears fall freely. It purged me of the anguish, and released me from the previous hurt I was experiencing.

There were two lessons I learned—Firstly, Satan does not care how he gets in, but he will try and try until a fissure is found, and then he will slip in as quickly as he can, take over for as long as he can, and hurt as many people as he can. It solidified in me an aspiration to pay attention to where I might be cracked. From the myriad of angles he could enter, I was confident he would attempt another disturbance.

Secondly, my family loved me, plain and simple. Period. End of story.

Chapter Twenty-Five

MY MOTHER'S PRAYER

It was the fourth of February and I had another painful afternoon that had me curled into a tight ball on the couch ... again. I remember begging Mom to heat the bean bag up, but it gave no relief. My pain levels had moved far past that treatment. Nothing worked—no matter what I did.

I had pulled completely inside of myself in an effort to survive the onslaught. The intensity of my agony was worse than all my previous experiences. This time it blasted me like electricity, throbbing with every thump of my heart, as if I were being electrocuted.

Mom kept pulling me back from the chasm I had fallen into, asking if I needed anything. I could not answer, but shook my head from side to side so slightly that she might have missed it. I glanced up at her ever so briefly; the look on her face was nothing short of panic. On a normal day, that might have frightened me. But on this day, I was so out of touch it did not even penetrate.

After hiding in pain for a long time, Mom got up and left the room. It was half past the hour. I closed my eyes and fell into the abyss of my situation. When I opened my eyes, I expected to see that an hour had passed, but only ten minutes had elapsed.

Within the next fifteen minutes or so, I began to gradually, but noticeably, feel a decline in the pain. I realized that Mom had not returned. I decided she was probably sick of having to watch my pain. I did not blame her. My heart slowed, my breathing eased, and I began to grow more peaceful.

Maybe Mom detected the alteration, because a few minutes later she emerged from the bedroom. She looked at me and our eyes connected for a time. That had not happened for several hours so she knew I was feeling better. She smiled a weary, relieved smile.

"Are you okay?" she asked as she walked toward me.

Looking up at her, I nodded in the affirmative. My energy had run out; I could not say a word.

"You look better," she said, kneeling next to the couch and reaching up to touch my hands.

I inhaled and forced a sentence. "Thought you'd given up on me."

"No," she stated, squeezing my hands. "I was praying. I think it worked."

My tired eyes met hers and appreciation settled over me. "Yes."

I wanted to say more, but I was far too drained. I never cherished my mother more than right then. She knew what to do. She taught me a valuable lesson that the Lord will come if you ask. It struck me again how much faith and love it took for my mother to pray away my pain. A few hours later, she gently suggested I stop taking the pain pills and the white willow bark at the same time. It made little sense to me and I said I would think about it.

~

The next morning was Sunday and Mike got up and dressed for church.

"You look very handsome," I said. I knew he would not dare say I looked beautiful just then. It had been nearly a month since I had curled my hair or applied any makeup to my face. Nonetheless, the look in his eyes told me he thought I was beautiful . . . regardless.

He smirked, "Thank you."

For a moment he said nothing, and then he took my hands in his and looked into my eyes.

"Do you mind if I tell everyone at church today?" he asked.

Every person, he was suggesting, was someone who loved and cared for me. But that would mean opening up my tiny circle of confidants to another four hundred people. Mike knew how I felt, but he waited for me to decide without putting any undue pressure on me. Then I finally came to a conclusion. "Okay. I think I'm ready," I said, still feeling a little tenuous about the situation.

"I think it will help to include them; more prayers are always better," he said.

He leaned in and hugged me carefully, holding me for a long time. I loved the feel of his body close to mine; his clean, shaven face next to my cheek and the smell of his skin.

"Okay then," he began, "I'll tell them." He stood, leaned over and kissed my face.

~

Mike returned three hours later to find me in my usual place on the couch.

"How are you feeling, Babe?" he asked as he reached out and touched me. The warmth from his hands always surprised me. I loved Mike; he knew how to get to my soul with something as simple as a touch.

"Better, actually," I said. I still felt crummy, but I did feel a little better.

Mike squeezed my hand. "Good, I'm glad to hear that."

Mom interjected from the kitchen. "Did you tell everyone what's going on?"

Mike looked up at her. "I did," he said, and then his gaze shifted back to me. "There sure are a lot of people who love you. Many were visibly shaken."

I almost choked on the bubble of air I swallowed. I felt my body jerk and lock into place like a Rubik's cube shifting into the winning position. "Four hundred people who love and care for me just began praying!" I heard myself say inside. I almost heard it click. "They love me!"

"Stacy was clearly crying," he said, "and somebody behind me literally sobbed out loud."

My lips were parted, seemingly ready to express the flood of emotion that was gushing in, but silence was the only sound. Suddenly I felt a very tangible warmth surrounding me. I closed my eyes, taking it in; I could feel their love. Mom interjected, taking Mike's attention away from my swiftly developing emotional state and the fact that tears were dripping from my eyes.

"What did you tell them?" Mom asked.

Mike glanced at her then back to me and said, "The bishop did not share what was going on with you, exactly, just that you were sick. Right after the meeting, nearly everyone in the room came up to me and asked what they could do to help. I found it odd that no one even asked *what* was wrong, they only offered their assistance." He turned and looked at me, adding, "I just asked them to pray." I could see a strange spark pass his eyes. Watching him release the load he had been carrying was a wonderful thing to witness. I realized that his burden of not telling anyone had been heavily weighing on him. I leaned in and said, "Thank you for telling them."

He chuckled, knowing I had not really wanted to tell. "You're welcome," he said as he leaned in closer to me.

I allowed a few tears to drip from my eyes into the fabric of his suit, and just lay there absorbing his love and feeling the prayers of our friends.

Chapter Twenty-Six

KNOWLEDGE IS POWER

I had been applying sea salt to my open wound for about two weeks. Every day the tumor came out of my body just a little farther. I took great assurance in that, but I was also suffering horrific, escalating pain as it attempted to detach itself from my body.

It was the middle of February. It had been six weeks since I had fallen so ill. I looked out the window and noticed it was snowing hard and I panicked a little. Don was scheduled to come to our house that day. I had no idea how comfortable he was in the snow. As if on cue, he called.

"I don't know if I can come today," Don said in an apologetic tone.

My heart sunk and started pounding against the interior wall of my chest. I had never had a panic attack before but was definitely on the verge of a full-scale mental assault. I stammered, "Oh! Please, please come!" in a tone that was desperate and completely foreign to my ears.

I felt bold, and reached up to put a hand over my lips attempting to stop any other brash or hasty comments. Don was doing me a favor. How could I be demanding? Silence hung on the line and I was afraid that maybe I had overstepped. Ideas of having to wait terrified me. If he did not come, I was certain I would shrivel and die on the spot. I needed him desperately, and I am positive that my voice exposed my need. Tears began to well in my eyes and I pressed my lips together, hoping they would not announce my mounting anxiety.

I turned away from the phone, leaving my ear pressed tight against the speaker. I closed my eyes and began praying that he would feel my need and just come. My hands grew hot and started to sweat. Don sensed exactly what was going on with me, showing how intuitive he was.

There was an immediate change in his tone as he said, "You know what? I'm going to come. It might take me a little longer to get there, but I'm coming."

An outpouring of gratitude engulfed me and the tears fell freely. They dropped against my shirt with an audible thump. Mike and Mom were watching intently, and Dad, who had come into town the day before, stepped into the room just as I was expressing my gratefulness to Don.

"Oh! Thank you so much! Thank you!" I said as I reached up wiping my cheek. "Thank you." I could barely contain myself.

Don chuckled and said, "I'll see you soon, Little Lady."

I hung up the phone and turned to look at Mom. She was crying too.

In my heart, I thanked God for answering my prayer. I smiled as big as I had in weeks, and immediately began praying that Don would arrive safely.

Sometime just after lunch, there was a knock on the front door. Mike opened it and happily greeted Don. He stepped in. I smiled. I had never been so happy to see anyone in my life.

Dad stepped forward and shook Don's hand and introduced himself. And then he introduced Mom. Don stepped toward the back of the couch where I was seated.

"Oh, it's good to see ya," he said with a soft country twang and tender quality he had not used with the others. The corners of his eyes creased gently as his smile softened into something that I can only describe as love. He reached out and took both of my hands in his, clasping them tenderly. Tears glistened in my eyes.

Taking one of my hands, I brushed the side of my hair. "I'm sorry, I'm not very presentable," I said apologetically. Then I tugged on my shirt and attempted to press out the wrinkles on the thigh of my yoga pants.

He laughed out loud, "Oh. You're so funny." The affectionate smile never left his face.

Mike offered him a seat. After sitting down in a chair directly in front of me, Don asked me to give him a brief rundown of my situation from beginning to end: what had gotten me to the doctor, and everything they did to me. So for the next few minutes, I detailed everything from the initial nine-month do-nothing period, to the testing, the biopsy and the mammograms.

As I spoke, the smile diminished and left Don's face. Concern was easily visible but he never interrupted me. He simply sat quietly absorbing every word.

When I finished and he began speaking, every previous thought I had was confirmed, and my heart sank to a profound place. I wanted to vomit.

"Biopsies led to the ulceration and fungal growth you're experiencing," he said. "That's just what they do. They disrupt your body's effort to encapsulate the problem and cause it to spread. You should never have a biopsy—ever," he said.

The way he had said *ever* rang in my ears. Instantly I was in mental agony, again, over my choice to have the biopsy. "But I didn't know!" I screamed at myself. My eyes glazed over and I kicked myself for my ignorance. Why did I give in? Why didn't I just follow my heart? It was a momentary decision that I perceived could easily have created a permanent and deadly change.

Gratefully, Don kept talking—it shook me out of my trance.

"Typically this type of explosion and infusion stays inside the body, but when they deposit material, such as that titanium clip or they administer radioactive particles in the way of contrast gels with MRIs or PET scans, it causes the growth," he explained.

My heart shattered and I heard myself speaking wildly and nervously about my choices. I tried to reason everything away and make him realize I did not usually go to doctors, but I was confused as to what to do.

He listened to my rant quietly and compassionately, letting me vent everything and throw it all down at his feet. When I stopped, he repelled my personal beating by changing the subject completely. For that I was thankful and it helped me let go of the self-disapproval.

Don looked at me and then toward my parents, saying, "I'm not sure your parents know anything about me, about what I do." His voice trailed off leaving the question hanging in the air.

I looked at Mom and nodded, "Yes, we've been talking about it a lot," I said as I turned my attention back to Don. He smiled and then began explaining himself to my parents anyway.

"I am the enemy in the pharmaceutical chemical camp, and yet they have me lecture at their symposiums four or five times a year. I think the number of oncologists who have quit their professions after coming to my lectures is up to forty-seven. So, they're coming around," he said smiling widely.

He looked at each of us in turn. His comments were hitting me hard. I began to develop an even stronger opinion about the medical industry. It made my blood boil to realize that I had unwittingly chosen to participate in activities that actually made my situation worse.

"Those doctors realized that no one dies of cancer—they die of the treatments. Then, when patients are finished with long chemical treatments, the doctors tell you the cancer is gone—until a few years later. Then they have to back up and say, 'Oh, there's a recurrence.' It's a vicious cycle that keeps going on and on and on ... *until you're gone.*"

The word *dead* registered in me with the accentuation of his final remark. I had read a lot about the statistics of traditional protocols. They were reasonable for a couple of years, ranging in the high nineties, but after five or ten years, the numbers dropped off like a rock to single digits.

Then Don said, "That is … *if* you have a good health care plan. If you don't, or you don't have any money, I've heard of people being sent home to die. I see and hear it all the time."

He continued telling a story about a famous football player's father-in-law who had dealt with cancer. "He was healed through natural protocols, and now he's just fine."

Don had my full attention. "We live in an era of such darkness and ignorance; people just don't know that they're victims of the wealthiest industry on the face of the earth. The medical industry is in existence to make money." He shrugged, "That's what they do."

Everything was spinning. Did they know? Did the doctors know what I was learning? Or were they turning a blind eye to reality?

"The body is the only thing that can heal itself. You have an immune system that will heal if it's supported properly. In this kind of situation, where the ulceration now has fungal growth … well, it sounds terrible but, the worse it gets, the better off you are because the body is pushing everything out. So, it's going to get worse before it gets better," he stated.

My mouth fell open just a little. I was not too excited for it to get worse, but I was astounded at the verbal evidence he was laying before me.

He looked at me, "Have you decided which route you're going to take; self-healing or medical?"

I did not hesitate. "Self-healing," I said. "It makes more sense and it just sounds right."

Mike interjected, "It's been so hard. We've just been so afraid. But it seems like most women just turn their lives over to the doctors."

It was good to hear Mike articulate those feelings. He never brought them up to me in private, so hearing them now settled my heart and put us both on the same page. He was looking for answers that would calm his heart as to the path I was insistent on taking.

"Exactly," Don responded. "They literally turn their lives over to them."

Then Don looked at me intensely. His eyes narrowed, he leaned forward and put his elbows on his knees. Then he zoned right in, "I'm glad you get this."

In a strange but profound way, Don was signing, sealing, and delivering the mental "okay" for me to accept the path I had chosen without reservation. He would be there to back me up, but it was up to me to remain solid and immoveable.

Then he sat up straight and looked at the others. "In their own medical literature it states that the number one cause of lumps in the breast is blocked drainage canals. The lymphatic nodes, which the breasts are full of, get blocked by bra straps. They cut off the circulation and honestly, shouldn't be worn unless you feel the need to do so in public. Not to mention that underwire bras often have radioactive wires in them. And then the number two cause is mammograms."

You could have heard a pin drop. The air in the room froze and everyone stopped breathing. My skin prickled at Don's comment and I cringed. I was pretty sure Mom was recoiling too. She had been faithful in getting her yearly check-up. For me, it was never something I did—except once. Then I never went again, until that fateful day the previous year. To me it never computed that irradiating your body was healthy, especially since it is common knowledge that radiation causes cancer.

I glanced over at Mom. The color had drained from her face. She had probably had twenty-plus mammograms in her life ... and breast cancer. She looked at me briefly and then turned her attention back to Don.

"The information is on the Internet. Anyone can find it, but like you said," he gestured toward Mike, "they're full of fear. Women run to the doctor and turn their lives over to them without much thought as to any other direction

146

they could go. And so, here you are now," he pointed at me, "the victim of that whole thing."

I flinched at the undesirable attention, my heart instantaneously leaping into my larynx.

"I'm just thankful you pulled back," he said.

Power and anger swelled within me. I knew he was speaking truth.

"Ancient scholars had studied the human body prudently, and when there were consistent results, they knew they had uncovered truth. That became words of wisdom and knowledge for future generations," he pronounced and then he reached up and adjusted the cowboy hat that sat atop his head. "The last shall be first and the first shall be last." He was quoting from the Bible; I wondered if he knew. "The very first symptoms you have will be the very last thing to go away. And the last thing you're experiencing will be the first to go away. It's a process of reversals. You are now in the stages of the very last of that process, so it'll start to clear up."

Mike spoke up again. "Most people would say that it's getting worse by the way it looks. How do you know it's getting better?"

Don went on to explain, "This is how healing takes place. If you start to get a fever it starts low, then goes high, and then back to low. It's like getting a cold or the flu; it gets worse before it gets better."

I could see the wheels turning as Dad opened his mouth to speak. And then he stopped, and then he opened it again as the words formulated. "Is there a benchmark in her case for how bad it's going to get, or is she at the top level now?"

"From the photo you sent, I think you're coming to the end of that," he responded.

It caused me to spark with what I had been seeing since putting salt on the lesion and I explained it to Don. "I feel like the salt is drawing liquid or something to the tumor because it's gotten a lot bigger, and it's gone quite dark.

I mean, before it was pink tissue, but now it's just dark and gross." I found myself describing the tumor in great detail. It probably turned my parent's stomach to hear it, but suddenly I just felt like I had to tell Don everything I was seeing.

He knew exactly what was happening and said very calmly as though it was no big deal, "It's dying. It will scab over and peel off."

I felt another explosion of confidence and caught myself smiling wide.

"So the tumor is dying?" Mike asked with a look of encouragement on his face.

"Yes," Don said.

That was it. There was no question; I could see it on his face. He knew what he was talking about. It made me feel powerful in my weakness, and I mentally embraced his vision for my future. I would heal; it might just take a little longer for the discomfort to pass. I had come this far and somehow I knew I could endure the rest of this journey. I began repeating positive affirmations to myself, "You can do this. You're almost there. It'll be over soon!"

"Tumors are the body's garbage cans," Don said. "They contain toxic residues. Your body will deconstruct it when the toxicity is gone, and it will travel out of your body. Truth is simple. When it gets complex, somebody is lying to you."

Don talked for another hour or more, teaching us everything from A to Z. I had settled into a peaceful ease, knowing without doubt that I was on the right path and that I could endure whatever else I had to. It felt so good to have my parents and Mike there learning. Now I was sure that my thoughts were theirs as well. They understood completely why I chose this road. So, even though they had been nothing but supportive, they were now a force of power behind me.

Before I knew it, the time was gone and Don had to go. I felt as though he had given me every key I needed to finish this thing, and I was profoundly grateful.

"Thank you so much for coming, Don," I said.

"It was my pleasure, Little Lady," he said with a crooked smile and a wink.

He moved to where he could reach me from the rear of the couch. "Yer gonna be just fine," he said with an exaggerated southern drawl. He reached around me, placing one hand on my shoulder and the other on my hair, and then he pressed his cheek next to mine.

I reached up with one hand and placed it on top of his hand. "Thank you," I whispered. I closed my eyes and let the love he was radiating saturate me. "Thank you so much."

He moved away just enough to speak directly into my ear, "Oh, I just appreciate being here face to face. It was important for us to do that," he replied quietly. He stepped back and patted my shoulders gently, and then moved toward the door. "Thanks for letting me come over," Don said as he looked at Mike. "I'm so proud of you. Love you guys."

I nearly laughed out loud at the intonation of his country voice.

Dad stepped forward and stuck his hand out to shake Don's. Don laughed as he stretched his arms out, rejecting the handshake. "I'm a hugger!" And with that, he took my father into a bear hug, and then Mom and Mike in turn.

Everyone was laughing as Don walked out the door and the earlier strain we had felt floated outside, too, leaving us light and happy and confident. I sighed as peace filled me.

Mike closed the door and I let myself replay his parting comments, "Yer gonna be just fine," and "Love you guys." How gracious he was. He had sacrificed for me, driving for an hour and a half in a newly laid blanket of snow—all because of the pleadings of a sick woman. My heart swelled; I knew I would be forever indebted to this man.

Chapter Twenty-Seven

SHE COULDN'T STAY FOREVER

Over the next few days I became unsettled. Although the weather was certainly a dark force just outside my windows, I was feeling something else—something more intense. I knew the peak of the mountain I was climbing was going to push me right to the edge of my limits. It was a strange thing to realize it was coming and I readied myself.

I don't remember it ever being so dark, cold, and miserable outside. The snow mounted and the grey skies conspired to keep me buried in shadows of drab, unforgiving gloom. My physical condition was deteriorating. Bad days were the norm, and worse days were becoming more frequent. I clung to Don's comments that the end of the tumor's progression was near.

~

Dad left and went back home. I knew it was hard for Mom to let him go again. They had hardly been separated during their many years of marriage, and I loathed being the reason they had to do it now. I could see how much the requirements of my life were wearing on her. It had been over a month since she had come. That same afternoon, she dropped a hint.

"At some point I'm going to have to go home," she said with faintness in her voice that I attributed to an attempt at softening the idea; she was planting a seed.

Instantaneously I was filled with terror. How would I eat? How would I function without her? Images filled me, and they were not pretty. I choked back an explosion that was developing in my throat and I expect my eyes widened with fear.

Mom saw it and said, "But only when you're ready. Just start thinking about it."

I breathed in to calm myself, but I also read into what she was really saying, which likely was something along the lines of how this whole situation was wearing her out to the point of illness. I felt horrible. I had already seen her fatigue. But she was the only one who could help me. At least that is what I believed at the time.

She stepped to me and gave me a gentle hug and then took her place at the end of the couch near my extended legs. As she often did, she picked my feet up, placed them on her lap and began rubbing them. I spoke a silent prayer and said, "Thank you, Heavenly Father, for my mother. I could never have done any of this without her."

As the day wore on, my need for pain pills fluctuated. Mom repeated her concerns about mixing the willow bark with the other meds I was taking.

"Let's try eliminating the willow bark all together today," she suggested. "It just seems to me that maybe the two things are not mixing well."

In some ways the thought scared me. What if the pain got worse without it? But instead of voicing my concerns, I shrugged and just said, "Okay."

Several hours went by. Pain was still my constant companion, but to my surprise, there were no episodes where I ended up crying, moaning, and curling into a tight ball. By that evening we were both convinced that Mom was on to something.

"You've had a pretty good day," she said encouragingly.

I nodded, "Yes. It's safe to say you figured out where the intense pain was coming from."

She smiled at me. I could see a release in her face I had not seen for a while. More often than not all I saw on her face was exhaustion. It did my heart good to see it, and gave me at least one afternoon with less pain than I had become accustomed to. Overall, it was the best day I had had in weeks.

~

February 22 was a Saturday. I had staggered through my usual morning routine; Mom had brought me breakfast in bed, then by noon I was curled up on the couch again.

"Your brother is coming today. He's going to take me out to lunch for my birthday," Mom announced.

"Crap!" I said in silence. "It's your birthday tomorrow! Dang it! I completely forgot! Some present; being trapped here with me!" A wave of frustration raced around me as I realized the repercussions. That was the first time I had ever forgotten her birthday. A bead of sweat began rolling down my temple as sadness closed in on me. "You forgot her birthday. How could you forget her birthday?" I asked, scolding myself.

But then another thought took over and I began to smile. She deserved the time away from my situation. She needed to get out, to forget about everything she had been dealing with. I was grateful and began thanking God for my brother and his insight into her situation.

I opened my mouth and spoke, "Well, that will be great. I'm sure you could use the sanity break from here."

"I think it will be nice," she said, not putting too much energy into it so I wouldn't feel left out of the fun. In reality, that was never a thought; I did not feel like going anywhere.

A few minutes later Mike came down the stairs. He had the day off and was expecting to spend most of his day caring for me.

"Good morning," he said enthusiastically to both of us.

"Morning," Mom replied.

I smiled and leaned back on the couch as Mike bent over to kiss my neck.

"How are you feeling?" he whispered.

"Mehhhh," I groaned. "Okay for now."

I took note that my attitude had slipped a little and I was giving into the negative emotions from the last several days. My pain levels had continued to ebb and flow, and although the willow bark was out of my regime, I still had notable swings in my pain levels, which wore on my psychological health as if someone had stacked multiple overweight books there. Until this time, I could not have even fathomed the depths that I was falling into, and how low the human body can actually go and not die.

Around twelve-thirty, my oldest brother arrived. On most days he was jovial and full of laughter, and filled the room with life and energy but, presumably because of my situation, he was holding back. He chuckled lightly and stepped into the room, handed Mom a huge butterfly balloon and a tight embrace. She was giggling. It was good to see her smile like that.

After releasing Mom, Brad shook Mike's hand, greeting him. Then he stepped around to the other side of the couch to me, almost cautiously. He pulled out a bar stool and turned it to face me. He said, "Hey, little sister, how are you?"

The look on his face was brooding and tense, and quite unfamiliar to me. At once I wondered if I looked as bad as I felt. I scooted into the back of the couch a little further, trying to sit taller. Maybe if I acted like I felt okay it would relax him. It did not really work. The jostling forced me to grimace and he saw it. His expression remained flat and unchanged.

I responded by saying, "Doing okay. How are you?"

It was a weak attempt to deflect the focus from me and shift it to him. Maybe it was not really the occasion to do that, but it had become my nature to redirect negative attention away from myself and minimize my own undesirable realities.

"Good. Good," he responded, almost awkwardly, but then he smiled.

I am not sure he knew what else to say, but his grin lit up the room and made me feel better. Several moments of uncomfortable silence slipped by until

Mom interjected comments about where they might go for lunch and questions about his family. Then they left.

Mom was gone for no more than two hours. I felt a little disappointed for her, thinking she needed way more time than that to recover from being my round-the-clock caregiver. And I felt even sadder about it because when she stepped back in, I was in the middle of one of my episodes. Silently, I was grateful that my brother had not walked her back in to witness it.

It took the majority of the afternoon to get back into some kind of balance, but even then it was not pain free. Every fiber of my being was fatigued. I could not have been any wearier if I had just scaled Kilimanjaro. Breathing was difficult, the fabric of my light cotton shirt weighed on my skin like a lead apron, blinking my eyes was forced and difficult, and I had a headache from the heaviness of my thin stringy hair. I began to question whether I was going to be able to continue to endure this energy-sucking experience. I was spent, wrung out and sapped. I felt like I had reached the end and could not take one step further.

Around nine o'clock that evening, I managed to rally a smidgen of energy and pulled myself off the couch, and lumbered up the stairs. Mom was cleaning the kitchen and Mike was sitting at the desk working on a project. I did not tell them what I was feeling or where I was going. I just got up and left. It took everything I had to get up the stairs and by the time I reached the top, I knew I had just enough energy to get myself to the bed or risk falling.

Sitting on the edge of the bed, I relaxed and lowered my chin. I contemplated how I was going to lay back onto the pillows: legs up first, or maybe put my elbow down on the mattress, but then that would mean bending. I breathed but did not move. My eyes closed and I took in another breath. The pain had been rising steadily for a long while, but as I sat there in the cool stillness of the room, it became quite acute and I heard myself cry out softly.

No more than thirty seconds later, Mike stepped through the doorway. "Are you okay?" he asked moving closer.

I groaned a little, "No, I am hurting about as badly as ever. I feel bad." It came out as a whisper.

If I had been the one standing there instead of Mike, I think I could have seen the pain with my naked eye. It hovered around me in shades of blood red and violent orange, burning my skin and encircling my body.

"Honey," Mike started with a level of despair I had not heard before. "Maybe it's time to go to the hospital." I knew by his comment, he could see what I felt.

Immediately my blood boiled and an energy I had not possessed before detonated, and then I lashed out at him. Even in my darkest moment I knew the Lord would fulfill his promise to me and in no uncertain terms I let Mike know it, too.

"No!" I said shooting an angry glanced in his direction with my eyes. "Stop it!" I demanded in a pathetically weak voice. "Just give me a blessing. It'll be fine."

Instantly I was humbled. How could I be so angry to the one person who loved me unconditionally? He was only trying to help. I felt a little ashamed about asking for a blessing in a fit of rage. Humility washed over me. "I'm sorry. I'm just not ready for that yet," I said.

Mike moved closer and kneeled at my feet and then touched my hand. It hurt, but I did not tell him that. "I love you," he said. "I'm sorry things are so hard and that you have to go through this."

Then he stood and gently laid his hands on my head. The words entered like warm golden oil that trickled into every corner of my body. It had been too many days since I had felt the calming influence of the Spirit of God. I relished the feeling.

He spoke of my being able to get through the night and that I would know what to do. When he finished, he helped me lay down, brought me the warm beanbag, and left me to sleep.

T

At around eight o'clock the next morning, I awoke and pulled myself to a sitting position. The pain intensified to an all-time high and I knew there was no more waiting. I was in trouble.

"Mike," I said weakly. He stirred only slightly so I repeated myself a little louder, which was not much since I felt so feeble. "Mike."

He came to full awareness fast. Rolled gently in my direction then said, "What? Are you okay?" It was loud and it startled me. It shocked him too.

"No," I said, trying to breathe between the waves of pain that were clutching me. "Get up. We're going to the hospital," I groaned, struggling to normalize my breath. The blessing Mike had given the night before had just been fulfilled. I had *gotten through* the night and I now knew what to do. I had to go to the hospital.

He sat straight up and jumped out of bed as fast as he could without shaking the mattress. If it had been any other situation than this, I might have laughed. He turned a full circle before realizing he needed to head into the closet for his clothing. I did not laugh.

I heard him in the closet rummaging for clothes. He came out in record time wearing jeans and a button-up shirt. He planted himself onto the chair that sat near the bedroom door and began putting his shoes on, and then asked, "Have you been in pain all night?"

"On and off. The blessing really helped and I did get some sleep, but it's time to go," I said, with as much force as I could. I rocked back and forth, moaning and holding my chest.

"Please go tell Mom what's going on," I said, hoping she would want to come with us.

"Okay," he replied, pulling the lace on his tennis shoe, "I'll be right back."

After he stepped out and headed downstairs, I reached for my phone, which was sitting on the nightstand. I found Don's phone number and texted him about the fact that I was about to go to the hospital. It felt like a huge defeat of everything I was trying to accomplish and I was a little unhappy that I had to break the news to him. But in all my discomfort, I knew I had to go.

Moments later, Mike was helping me get up and steadying me as we walked down the stairs. Mom was already dressed in her coat and ready to go. I had slept in my yoga pants and one of Mike's cotton shirts. All I needed was my coat and boots, which Mom helped me slip into.

Mike held my arm as I hobbled to the door. Mom mentioned that Dad was coming for her birthday, which was that very day. I cringed. We were going to the hospital on her birthday. "I couldn't catch him before he left to tell him what's happening," she said, "so I wrote a note to stick on the outside of the front door."

I remember seeing the yellow post-it on our way out and hoped that Dad would see it, too.

As Mike put me into the front seat, I let out a horrible, pain-filled cry. As Mike drove I felt every bump, every rock, every crack, every curve, and every hill.

The drive took thirty minutes, but it went by in a blur to me. I was so intently focused on not moving that I barely noticed anything. I was aware of Mom's hands tightly gripping each of my shoulders and pinning them to the back of the seat. Appreciation filled me for her efforts because both my hands were busy trying to hold my body still. I cried and moaned at every movement and Mike kept apologizing as he tried to minimize the unsteadiness of the car ride.

It struck me that the last time I had been away from the house it had been the fourth of January. Today was the twenty-third of February—a Sunday, and Mom's birthday.

Chapter Twenty-Eight

ANOTHER PROPOSAL OF DEATH

We arrived at the hospital, taking the liberty of parking directly in front of the Emergency Room entrance. Mike got out and rushed to the passenger side of the car and Mom moved to my side as soon as some unknown person with a wheelchair came out and assisted me out of the car.

The time it took to check in probably amounted to about twenty minutes, but it felt like hours. The pain had escalated to a point that I could barely breathe. I caught myself rocking back and forth like a child trying to answer the myriad of ridiculous questions they were asking: my address, who my insurance carrier was, my telephone number. I answered the best I could, but in truth I was screaming at them to get me some help—but they never heard it pass from my lips.

Domination and mindset had become the name of the game regarding the pain. But in this situation, where I was forced to place my attention on other matters, the pain escalated violently like internal punctures of a thousand needles working their way to the surface from the inside out. Almost as quickly as I processed their questions and answered them, I would find myself pulling back into a frenzied mental state where I worked to regulate my body. It was exhausting.

My ears perked at moaning sounds that stabbed the air around me, at first they seemed far away and distant, as if they belonged to some patient down a corridor who was in horrible agony, and then I realized they were not the noises from another patient in the ER—they were coming from me. If I had been on the outside observing, the sight would have crushed me to tears.

Before long they wheeled me into a small, dark room, helped me take my coat off and lay me onto a bed. After a little while, someone entered and announced to Mike and Mom that they were taking me to run some tests. Most of what happened during that time was pretty hazy to my memory, but I recall being delivered back to my ER room and lying in the dark—mentally and physically drained—for quite some time before anyone else came in.

It was all I could do to manage the pain while we waited. The pain seethed in and squeezed tight as though someone had rolled me up in a sheet and then began twisting it tighter and tighter until I thought I might explode from the pressure. Sounds were muted but constant. Buzzers, bells, and a heart monitor beeped nearby. I heard Mike and Mom talking quietly and recounting the ride down the icy canyon road.

There were so many voices passing by my doorway, and footsteps shuffling back and forth on the linoleum floor. It all became a distorted and confusing mess, swallowed up by the fact that I was completely engrossed in regulating the pain.

I blinked as I heard a person entering my room. I saw a figure standing in the doorway with a folder. I heard another person enter and move to the side of my bed. I blinked again and saw a young woman in scrubs inserting a needle into an IV that I had not realized was sticking out of my arm. It burned as it entered my veins.

The woman in the doorway was flipping layers of papers on her clipboard and mumbling to herself, and then she abruptly introduced herself as Dr. Karen Louder. Her voice startled me and I opened my eyes again. She announced that she had read over my file and what Dr. Howard had said the previous December. I flashed back momentarily to his comment about dying. I wondered if he were right.

Then I reconnected with Dr. Louder's voice. It was full of scorn that I had not heard from many people in my life before now.

"You could die today," she said in a rather matter-of-fact tone. "You could die before the day is out, actually, or tomorrow, or in a few days!"

I tried to see who would be audacious enough to make such a venomous announcement in the presence of my mother. Her comments hit me like the cold surge of sea water after an iceberg broke and fell; they were brash and cold-hearted and thoughtless.

In my mind I was screaming, "What? Who the heck are you? How dare you talk about me that way in front of my mother and husband!"

My hair pressed back down into the pillow with a soft thud. A million things raced through me, "I might die today? I don't feel like I'm that close to death. It's just a lot of pain. Can't you stop the pain? Give me something for the pain! It would really mess things up if I died. Isn't it Mom's birthday today? Where's Dad … is he still on the road driving down from Idaho? What if I do die?"

I looked over at Mom who was crying. In a second I forgot the pain and was furious! I attempted to breath in enough air to tell that woman what I thought about her callousness, but nothing happened. I could not formulate the words. My body was in complete management of my physical power and the fighting spirit inside of me had nothing to give. There was no energy for movement or conversation, only the barest of necessities—like breathing.

"Maybe I am dying," I thought.

I looked at Mike whose face had drained of all its color and tears dripped from his eyes, hitting the knee of his jeans. The nurse, who had come in earlier, was looking at the floor, obviously uncomfortable with the comments being thrown about so cruelly.

It felt like I were having an out-of-body experience. My fury was transcendent at that time, but there was nothing I could do; my frame would not move. If I could have, I would have gotten off the bed and punched Dr. Louder in the mouth!

She rattled on for quite a while. I heard her say something about how the tumor was dead. "What?" I responded wordlessly, "The tumor is dead? I did it! It's dead!" In all the vehemence I felt, it instantly vanished in the comprehension of that comment. If I could have, I would have smiled.

I felt elated, and a powerful smugness filled me. It also became apparent that the syringe that had been discharged into my veins earlier was pain medication and it was beginning to work, I felt more coherent.

Dr. Louder continued speaking, "Her blood has gone septic from the dead tumor; it's decomposing inside of her body and causing sepsis in her blood," she said. "So some decisions have to be made immediately."

Dr. Louder wanted to start me on antibiotics. Mike stood and walked over to me. Leaning in, he tried to discuss it with me. I had difficulty wrapping my mind around the questions but, strangely, I recognized the fact that he was still giving me all the power to make my own decisions. That amazed me. I nodded, agreeing to the antibiotics.

Closing my eyes, I relaxed and let the pain medication take over. I relished in the fact that my lungs were expanding more fully than they had in days. My body was exhausted. I breathed deep again. It felt good, and in some perplexing way, I was happy. The tumor was dead!

~

Dad, who was completely unaware of the goings on at the hospital, was driving into town. I am certain he expected to arrive, find us all at the house, and spend the day with my Mother for her birthday. But what he found was a note.

Mom had written, "Please call me from Alicia's house phone."

She had not written anything else for fear that it would alarm him and he would drive to the hospital frantic, potentially endangering himself and others.

As he related it later, he found the note, let it settle in for a few minutes, and then he prayed. A strong and profound impression came to him and he just knew that he was needed at the hospital.

Dr. Louder left my room and moments later Dad stepped in. I opened my eyes as he reached down and touched Mom's leg. She was seated near the door. He smiled at her. Mom looked broken and tired.

He stepped close to me and picked up my hand. Ease filled my heart; knowing he was near brought a sense of calm. For a few minutes I was a little girl again being soothed from a fall off of my bicycle. It was as if my spirit connected with his. The energy flowed from him into me like a current of love, relaxing and lulling me to sleep for a time.

I have no remembrance of how much time had passed, but after I awoke the doctor came back into my room and suggested that I be admitted to the hospital. Mike looked at me. I nodded in agreement. Shortly after that, I was wheeled to a room on the third floor.

As we entered, Mom and Dad moved to the far end of the room and sat on a small couch. Mike stepped close to my side and asked if I wanted him to call the kids.

"Yes," I said, half slurring the word. "They need to know what's going on." The drugs were working. The pain was diminished substantially but I felt pretty dozy. I decided it was acceptable in contrast to the alternative.

Each of my children came that night, and although I do not recall the details of their visits, I was aware of their presence, which filled me with comfort.

Chapter Twenty-Nine

BALANCING ACCEPTANCE AND REJECTION

By the next morning I felt a lot better. The combination of a decent night's sleep and the reduced pain allowed me to feel somewhat revitalized. It was my first full night's sleep in more than six weeks. Sometime before breakfast arrived, Dr. Steven Browning came in. I had never met him before, but I recalled his name as the surgeon who worked in the same office with Dr. Howard. Dr. Howard had mentioned him to me and that he was no longer taking new patients, so it struck me odd that he was even in my room.

He was a tall man, maybe six feet or more, with striking blue eyes and light hair that was touched with grey. He had a gentleness about him that I had not seen in any of the specialists I had met to this point. It was refreshing. When he spoke, his voice was soft and kind, and he smiled, which took me completely by surprise. I immediately felt at ease.

He reported the findings of my initial testing—a CAT scan and blood work. The tumor was indeed dead, but the fact that it was decomposing and leaching into my body meant it had to come out. I thought to myself, "This is the *procedure* mentioned in my blessing."

"The only way I can see getting it out is doing a mastectomy," Dr. Browning said.

I was taken aback but, oddly, I did not feel nervous or scared, or any type of emotion you might expect with such a conversation.

I did not give him an answer right away; instead I said, "Okay, let me think about it."

Since he was talking about doing the procedure in a day or two, I had time to think. I was no longer in danger of dying from the sepsis. It also gave me time to call Don, and discuss options with Mike. After every other medical person I had experienced, I was not going to just give in and turn my life over to someone without analyzing the facts and praying about it. After all, I had turned my life over to God up to this point, why just give away my power now?

"Fair enough," Dr. Browning responded. "I'd like to order a PET scan as well. It will show if the cancer has spread to any other part of your body."

"Let me think about it, and get back to you on that," I replied.

I think he was a little surprised by my unwillingness to jump in immediately, but his reactions were exactly what I would have wanted—calmness and acceptance of the fact that I was going to make my own decisions.

"All right," he said. "If you decide today, let the nurse know. I'll be back tomorrow morning to discuss things with you."

I appreciated the fact that he was not shoving his opinions down my throat; he was letting me decide. It made all the difference in my respect for him, and willingness to listen to his advice.

A nurse, who had followed Dr. Browning in, lingered after he walked out. She asked if I had any questions.

"Yes, I would like to talk to someone about the PET scan and what that entails," I said.

She quickly wrote down a phone number and gave it to me. My aim was to find out what dangers, if any, were associated with the test. I did not get a chance to call, however, because there was another doctor stepping in my doorway just as she was leaving.

"Hello," he said without looking at me. "I'm Dr. Hillary, an oncologist here at the hospital."

The pleasant feelings I had when Dr. Browning was in the room faded and were replaced by an uneasiness that is difficult to describe, but I sensed something negative so I paid attention.

"I'm here to discuss chemotherapy and radiation treatment," he started.

"No. I'm not interested in that," I said. "Thanks."

He looked shocked that I would even dare say such a thing—disbelieving, in fact. What struck me was that he never made eye contact. He sort of shuffled his feet, buried his hands in his pockets, and looked at his shoes. I studied the body language; he was uncomfortable.

"I see. Well, I'll stop back tomorrow," he said, and then turned and left.

I looked at Mike. "That was weird," I said.

"Yes … very," Mike said and then he continued, changing the subject, "You need to text Don. He's been sending messages all afternoon. He's really worried about you. Plus, he needs to know what Dr. Browning is recommending."

I sent a text to Don to let him know I needed to talk to him, and could he please call? Two minutes later my phone rang. I answered it and put it on speaker so Mike could hear.

"I am so glad you texted. I've been worried sick!" Don said with a lot of emotion in his voice.

"Me too," I said, feeling relieved that he called so quickly. I needed his perspective. "The surgeon was here a few minutes ago and is suggesting a mastectomy. I don't think there is any way around it at this point."

"What do you think about what he said, Mike?" Don asked, shifting his attention.

"It seems the only thing to do, unless you have any other ideas," Mike replied.

I so appreciated Mike's openness and continued support of my desire to live holistically, even in this situation where it did not seem that there was a viable option for my chosen path.

"Under normal circumstances, I would never recommend surgery, but under these circumstances I agree that it's probably the best course of action," Don said.

I interjected into the conversation saying, "Oh, and this oncologist came …"

Before I could even finish Don interrupted me and said, "*No chemotherapy or radiation—ever! We will do what we need to after the surgery to heal your body, but don't do the poison and burn!*"

His voice was resolute and strong, stronger, in fact, than any time previously.

I laughed, something not done in weeks. "I knew you were going to say that," I said. "I already told him I wasn't interested."

"Good girl," he said. I could hear the relief in his voice. "You text me after the surgery, when you're up to it, and let's chat again."

"I will for sure," I said, running the words together as though my tongue were swollen. "If the doctor is able to clear his schedule, it'll most likely be Wednesday morning."

Mom and Dad and Mike and I discussed everything for quite a while. Then Mom and Dad excused themselves to go out and get a bite to eat. Mike took the occasion to kneel next to my bed and offer a prayer, asking if surgery were the right thing to do. By the time "amen" was said, we both knew. "Well, okay. I guess its surgery then."

"Okay," Mike responded solemnly.

Mike stood and said he would let the nurse know of our decision. As he stepped to the door, he reached for the handle and then turned and looked at me.

Behind the slight smile on his face I could see peace, the confidence that only a message from heaven could have brought.

While he was gone, I closed my eyes and prayed, "Thank you, Heavenly Father, for bringing me to this point where I can finally feel settled and calm ... and even peaceful. I am ready now, ready to accept the *procedure*."

My heart sank a little as I contemplated the fact that I likely could have had a smaller procedure done a year ago when I was first diagnosed. "No!" I said to myself as I jerked my mind away from the regret. "Just be grateful."

"I am grateful," I whispered audibly. "Thank you for bringing me peace today, thank you for letting me learn, thank you for being right here when I've needed you most. I love you."

Warmth blanketed me as I closed my eyes, dozing off for a while.

~

A while later I awoke to see Mike was sitting near the window. Suddenly my nurse Allie came bounding in. "I don't know how you did it, but you have about the best surgical team there is around here. Everyone is talking about it and is amazed. You'll be in the best hands!"

"Really?" I asked questioningly.

She nodded and spoke rapidly and excitedly. "Yes! I've worked with Dr. Browning before. I used to be an ER nurse. Trust me, he'll do whatever it takes to do things right. He's amazing. I'm so excited that he's the one you have for your surgeon. Everyone says he's the best, even all the other doctors. Isn't that great?" she asked, and then without waiting for my response she continued, "I don't think you'll be disappointed; he does very meticulous work. And everyone else in the team is the best of the best, from the anesthesiologist to the nurses. I just can't believe it! It doesn't happen very often around here, so you are really lucky."

Her declaration settled within me—not as any kind of luck, but as the blessing that it was. I remembered Dr. Howard's declaration about Dr. Browning not taking on new patients. All I could do was smile, knowing full well who put the team together. Here I was, with apparently the best lineup available in the region. There was no doubt how it all happened. I looked toward the ceiling and whispered, "Thank you."

Chapter Thirty

THE THIRD TIME IS NOT THE CHARM

Dr. Browning came in the next morning around ten.

"Good morning. How are you feeling?" he asked, standing straight.

"Doing much better than the last few days, thank you," I said sluggishly.

My speech was still sloppy from the medication. It annoyed me, but at least I was coherent enough to make decisions. I was happy about that.

"Good, I'm glad you're feeling better. The medication is working all right?"

"Yes," I said. "Maybe too good." I reached up and wiped at the saliva forming at the corners of my lips.

He chuckled and said, "I'm glad to hear that. What did you decide about surgery?"

"We're going to go ahead with that," I responded. "And if you're still able to clear your schedule, it makes more sense to do it tomorrow than to wait until Friday."

"I agree. I already cleared it just in case," he said as he took a step closer to me. "The surgery is going to be a bit of a challenge. The PET scan confirms that the tumor is dead, but it's large and the skin will be difficult to close after I get it out, but I think everything will go fine. Oh, and Dr. Hillary will be in later to give you the full results of the PET scan."

Inside I cringed and the hair on the back of my neck stood up. I did *not* want to see Dr. Hillary again. I wondered what more he could add to what Dr.

Browning had just said. The tumor was dead. "What more did I need to know?" I wondered. Consoling myself about his expected return I reasoned, "If there is actually more to know, that is the *only* reason Dr. Hillary would be allowed back into my room." He had rubbed me wrong on his first visit and I was not really interested in the dark feelings again.

Dr. Browning continued, "There is a slight chance that one lymph node is affected. It showed some abnormality on the scan, but there was nothing else; no cancer anywhere in your body."

I smiled and began talking inside to myself. "You did it, Alicia!" And then I audibly stated, "If you don't absolutely have to take that lymph node, please leave it," I said firmly.

I knew that removing any of the lymphatic system would leave me susceptible to numerous other possible health issues down the road, and I did not want them touched.

He looked at me and saw the seriousness in my eyes. "I won't take anything I don't have to," he said, dropping his chin to connect eye to eye with me. There was sincerity in his eyes that told me he was trustworthy. From that moment, I believed he was in fact sent by God to help me.

"Okay then," Dr. Browning said, "I'll see you in the morning."

It hit me hard just after he left the room that the Lord was coming through with all the blessings he promised me. I knew it. I felt it. I believed it.

~

As the day wore on, Mom and Dad, who had been there since nine that morning, decided to go get lunch; it was their fifty-ninth wedding anniversary.

"You have to go," I said emphatically. "You deserve an afternoon out."

As they stepped toward the door, Mom squeezed my toes under the blanket and winked.

A few minutes after that, Mike mentioned he was hungry, too. "Will you be okay if I go get some food?" he asked.

I smiled at the concerned look on his face. "Yes, I'll be fine."

Mike had slept at the hospital for two nights on an unpleasantly-hard foldout bed that doubled as the couch during the day. His devotion and concern for me was impressive, and I appreciated it more than he knew. There was something very comforting in the fact that he was just there if I needed him.

"I'll be back in about a half an hour," he said as he bent over and kissed me softly.

"Okay," I smiled, blinking slowly and forcing my eyes open. "I'll be here."

He laughed at my attempt at humor then walked out the door. I closed my eyes and smiled, and then began musing about what life would be like when I healed completely.

Moments later, Dr. Hillary walked in, interrupting my meditation. I felt uneasy.

"Hello there," he started. The sound in his voice was flowery and light. I was surprised to see that he was actually looking at me.

"Good morning," I said quietly and cautiously, gathering my wits about me.

"So I hear you're going to have surgery in the morning," he commented, lifting his chin and looking almost happy, except without the smile. His eyes told the story.

"Yes," I said blandly. I did not want to get into a conversation about it.

I watched him closely, trying to read him, and annoyed that he had even been told about the surgery since he would not be involved in my situation. All I wanted were the test results.

He pulled his hands out of his pockets and put one of them on his hip, letting the other fall to his side, and then he began shifting his weight nervously back and forth.

Then he began to lie to me.

His right hand came up and began swirling about in almost dance-like form. "We don't know exactly where the cancer has gone. It could be deep in your muscles or even into the bones," he said while he looked around the room instead of at me. "We're just not sure," he stated.

A heat rash flushed across my chest. I knew it. I could feel it even though I could not see it due to the high-necked hospital gown. He's lying. I could feel my ears get hot. He might have noticed the tightness of my jawline, or the darkening of my eyes, if he had bothered to actually look and connect with me, but he did not; that was not his agenda.

"So, chemotherapy will be an important factor after surgery," he said as he reached up and scratched the side of his mouth. His voice trailed off.

"No, I already told you I was not going to do that."

The head of my bed was raised just enough that I could easily see his whole body. For effect, I dropped my chin and zoned directly into him, willing him to make eye contact with me.

He turned, almost sheepishly and glanced at me. I expect he noted that I had a solid lock on him—drugs or not. His eyes were wide, I could hear his breathing quicken, and his mouth hung open just far enough that I knew exactly what he was thinking. He was in shock. I doubt he had ever had anyone turn him down so flatly. He almost looked like he had been caught with his hand in the proverbial cookie jar. I read him like a book.

He dropped his eyes again and cleared his throat, and then he squared his shoulders and looked at me straight on. He squinted somewhat as he looked toward the window and then back at me again. His hands pushed a little deeper into his pockets making the fists he was clenching easily detectable. Then he spoke. It was not what I expected him to say, but it was powerful and stabbed into me like a double-edged sword, "You know you're going to die, don't you?"

"That was bold," I thought, but I said nothing, initially. I just stared back at him with fire in my eyes. He looked at the floor again and shook his head from side to side. I could see his jaw thicken as he clamped his teeth down hard. The air around him seemed poisonous and murky, as if something dark and indiscernible was inside him, ready to explode.

My mind was in a fury, and I think he finally realized it when I said, "I already told you, I don't intend to do chemotherapy." He looked at me briefly and said, "I see … well, good luck to you then." Then he spun on his heels and stomped out of the room like an angry teenager.

I closed my eyes and muttered a prayer of thankfulness to Heavenly Father. The warmth I had come to love flooded over me, filling the room with light and peace.

Mike came walking back into the room about ten minutes later. When I told him about my experience with Dr. Hillary, he said, "Wow that was nervy. Sounds like you sent him packing though. Makes you wonder if he needed a new car or something."

"Whatever it was, it was wrong. He should be ashamed of himself," I said angrily. "When I get done with all of this, someone is going to hear about it."

Mom and Dad came walking back a few minutes later.

"You've had your fair share of bad doctors, haven't you?" Mom said as her brow creased in disbelief. "I can hardly believe that. What is that now, three?"

I knew she was referring to the number of medical professionals who had predicted an early demise for me and were anything but professional with me.

"Yes," I said. "Three out of the four specialists I've seen. Those are some pretty bad odds; makes me wonder about the rest of them out there."

I did not include Dr. Browning in that tally. He was capable and proficient and I trusted him—mostly because of the good feelings I had felt when he was around. I held him in high regard and trusted that he would do his best during surgery.

That night I told Mike to go home and get some uninterrupted rest. He asked me if I were sure, to which I told him, "Yes, as long as you are back before I leave for surgery." He stayed that evening until ten.

Chapter Thirty-One

THE PROCEDURE

The sun had just cracked over the mountains to the east when a nurse stepped in to administer some medication. It was hard for me to accept that it was necessary. It ran so contrary to what I had come to believe, but I was grateful. I had to admit that there was a definite place for pain medication. The obvious effects I could detect from the particular medication they had been giving me were some vertigo and slurred speech. I knew that after I finished my prescriptions, Don and I would do whatever it took to cleanse my body from any residual toxins from the medications.

Mike arrived around nine. Thirty minutes later a young orderly came into my room. His badge read "Noah." He was tall and lanky, and had a spark in his eyes. He announced that he was there to take me to surgery. Mike stepped to the bed and helped me stand. Noah slid the wheelchair beneath me and we rolled toward the door.

"I'll see you soon," Mike said as we bounced a little heavily across the threshold. I moaned.

"Oh, sorry!" Noah said, "I'll be a little more cautious on the bumps." He smiled and asked my name and then asked, "Well, Alicia, do you like to drive fast?"

"In my car, or in this chair?" I quizzed. I was a little nervous about his question, but soon realized that the pain medication made the trip in the wheelchair quite bearable.

"Well, you strike me as someone who loves to drive fast in a car, but I was referring to the chair."

I chuckled and tightened my grip on the arms of the chair. "Wheel away driver," I said as he shifted into a slightly higher gear.

As we approached the elevator, Noah literally skidded to a stop, his shoes dragging a bit on the short-carpeted floor. He leaned out, pushed the down-arrow button and then stepped back to wait for the doors to open.

"I'm pretty new. If I do a good job and work quickly, maybe they'll keep me around a while," he stated through a straight, white smile. I wondered if that included getting me safely to the operating room.

Our trip to surgery took just a little longer than planned, however, because Noah wheeled me off the elevator onto the first floor. Ten seconds into our short journey, he realized his mistake. We made a U-turn and got right back on the elevator.

"Sorry about that. I'm still learning my way around," he explained apologetically.

I smiled. "No worries," I said, actually beginning to feel a little frustrated and nervous at his haphazardness. His fast pace and neglect of detail filled my heart with anxiety and the reality of what I was about to undergo hit me like a snowball in the face.

We stopped on the correct floor the next time and exited the elevator. Noah pushed the wheelchair until we came to a small room with a gurney bed. There was no door, only an ugly brown and gold curtain. A nurse greeted me and thanked Noah, who hurried away. I breathed a sigh of relief as a second nurse stepped into the room. The two of them helped me stand and move onto the gurney. It shocked me how wobbly I felt. It had been less than ten minutes since I had left my room and I had not felt as dopey as I did just then.

The nursed asked me a question, which I heard, but it sounded as if it came from another room, foggy and detached. I did not answer her.

She asked again, "Alicia, how are you feeling?"

It came clear that time, "Okay, considering all things," I said as they laid me back on the pillow. I closed my eyes, mentally disappearing.

Someone came into the room and spoke to the nurse, and then moved across the room. Touching my hand he said, "Alicia, good morning. I'm Dr. Woods; I'll be your anesthesiologist. We'll get started in just a few minutes."

I opened my eyes and caught a quick look at him as he moved to the other side of the bed. He had on green scrubs and a surgical cap secured to the top of his head, and grey hair sticking out from the bottom. There was a mask tied loosely around his neck on one end and dangling freely across his upper chest on the other. His shoes were enclosed in stretchy blue covers that made his steps silent as he walked.

As he moved past the curtain doorway, Dr. Browning came around it and walked toward me. He touched my arm and said, "Good morning, Alicia. Are you ready?"

I blinked. "The question is, are you?" I joked, smiling.

"I'm always ready," he stated.

"That was the right answer," I said. "Thank you."

"Everything is going to work out just fine," he said confidently. "Let's get you into surgery."

At that, he moved to the top of my bed and pushed me out the doorway. Above me the fluorescent lights passed by as we rolled down a long hallway, and then we turned a corner and passed through a doorway with large glass windows in them. It struck me odd that there were windows where anyone could look in during my surgery and see what was going on. I felt uncomfortable with the idea since I knew that everything private and sacred to me would be pretty much exposed.

Inside the room there were four or five people waiting. Dr. Browning moved me close to the table that stood in the middle and asked, "Alicia, do you think you can stand and move from the gurney to the table, or would you like us to use a roller to move you over?"

"This medication is making me pretty shaky," I said, hardly feeling my legs at all. "You'd better use the roller."

I felt myself being slid across to the table, and then bam, I was out. The next thing I knew, someone was tapping my hand and calling my name.

"Alicia. It's time to wake up. Can you open your eyes for me? Alicia? Come on, you can do it, open your eyes."

My eyes fluttered, but I could not open them. Around me there were many voices saying much the same thing. I perceived they were talking to other patients who had just gotten out of surgery, too. I suddenly felt like I was part of a herd of cattle and although I could not open my eyes and see what was happening, I distinctly remember feeling embarrassed to be in such a place—like one of a hundred others that day being rolled through on a conveyer belt.

The nurse tapped my hand again. "Alicia? Can you open your eyes?"

I tried, but they only fluttered again.

"She's ready," The nurse said to someone as I felt my bed move. I was being rolled somewhere, but I could not open my eyes, no matter how hard I tried.

Suddenly my mind went wild. I envisioned everything from aliens to the Stepford Wives[3]—everything but reality. I was instantly terrified as my heart began racing, and I wondered where Mike was.

From off in the distance, I suddenly heard him. "Oh, there she is," he said. I still could not open my eyes, but in an instant my concerns and fears were washed away because of his voice, and I knew that everything was going to be all

---

[3]*The Stepford Wives* is a 1972 satirical thriller novel by Ira Levin.

right. We turned a corner and I realized I was in my room. Mom and Dad were there, which added to my feelings of safety.

A few unfamiliar voices surrounded me and lifted me into my bed via a blanket that lay beneath me, and then I heard the gurney shake as it hit the door on its way out. A nurse came in and said, "They said she's having a hard time waking up, so talk to her."

I tried to form a few words, but all I got out was a whispered, "Wow." But to Mike's ears it probably sounded more like a shallow puff of air. I heard him laugh at my communication attempt. "It's okay honey; you don't have to talk. Just try and open your eyes."

It was not really a surprise that the medication had such a strong effect on me. I had always been sensitive to medications and stimulants. Once, several years before, I had taken a few caffeine-filled pain pills for a massive headache. For nearly two hours my hands shook violently as if I had some sort of physical disorder.

About an hour later I was feeling better, but was still not completely articulate. I drew a complete blank about the entire surgical experience, and the lingering medications left me feeling bleary. In other ways, I was grateful that I could not recall anything yet.

I decided it was a good thing I trusted my surgeon because under the circumstances, I was in as vulnerable a position as I had ever been in my life.

Shortly afterward, Dr. Browning came in to see how I was doing.

"Mike could you help me raise the bed a little?" I asked as he did so. "So ... how did it go?" I asked, turning my attention to Dr. Browning.

"Everything went really well. I was concerned we wouldn't be able to close completely, but I managed to get it done. Everything looks good, in fact, much better than I expected. The margins were clear. Frankly, I'm surprised that it didn't spread."

Inside I screamed, "Ha! I know why!" But the only thing I said was, "Oh, that's good."

Then he continued, "You did, however, lose a lot of blood, which has made you anemic. Will you accept a blood transfusion?" he asked.

"No," I said, surprised that I was coherent enough to even make that decision. "I'd rather not." Somewhere in my heart I knew that Don would remind me how to get my blood count back up, but at that moment it completely eluded me.

"Well, can we at least give you some iron?" Dr. Browning quizzed.

"Yes, that'll be fine," I answered, surprised at my ability to comprehend and respond.

At that he left to give the orders to the nurse. I turned to Mike and asked if he would hand my phone to me. He did so, and I sent Don a message, asking him to call when he had a chance.

A little while later my phone rang. I could see by the caller ID that it was him. I answered it and then put it on speaker so we could all hear.

"How are you feeling?" he asked.

"A bit fuzzy, but okay. Thank you," I said.

I remembered what Dr. Browning said about my being anemic and told Don that I had refused the blood transfusion and asked what I should do instead.

"Good girl," he said enthusiastically. "That was the right choice." Then he proceeded to remind me about raw eggs and organic grape juice. "And now that you're finished with all of this, no more tests, no more scans!" he said firmly. I knew what he meant. This was not a situation I wanted to revisit again, ever.

Chapter Thirty-Two

GRAPE JUICE, EGGS AND ANGELS

It was late afternoon the day of my surgery when Mike, Mom and Dad decided to leave the hospital to get some lunch, and buy eggs and grape juice for me.

I was hoping to get a short nap, but not ten minutes later, Dr. Hillary stepped in.

If my inward contemplations had exhibited themselves externally, he would have seen me roll my eyes, but in reality I stayed cool on the outside.

"Hello," he said looking briefly at me, then admired his ever-loved brown loafers again.

My body stiffened and I responded coolly, "Hello."

"I just wanted to come and see how things went with your surgery and if you were ready to talk about treatment options," he said. He bounced on his toes and then shuffled his feet from side to side, dragging them back and forth across the linoleum as if he were on a beach drawing pictures in the sand with his toes. And, as was usual, he avoided any and all eye contact.

"Dr. Hillary, I told you I was not going to do that," I said, densely.

The look on his face changed from awkwardly encouraged, to angry bewilderment. He glanced at me to see if I were serious, and then back at his shoes. I was serious and he saw it.

I could not comprehend his persistence. Was he incapable of taking "no" for an answer? Then it occurred to me that his appearance in my room on the day of my surgery may have been premeditated—I had just awakened from being drugged … and he knew it. I grew more and more furious the more I thought about it. How was it that every single time my family left, he appeared? I wondered and it did not sit well with me. It seemed calculated.

When he spoke next he sounded like a whiney child asking relentlessly for a lollypop. "Well, what can I do for you then?" he said, scowling a bit out of spite. Both of his arms came up, flapping briefly like a bird. I half expected him to stamp his feet and clench his fists.

"Nothing," I said with as much energy as I could, which under the circumstances was not much. I cannot imagine the look on my face left any question however.

I felt my face getting hot. I was not budging and thought maybe he finally understood.

"Well then, I'll leave you alone," he said as he turned and left rather abruptly.

~

When Mike and my parents returned, it took nearly two hours, and a lot of discussion to calm down enough to let go of the obstinate Dr. Hillary.

"He's like a gnat that won't go away no matter how many times you swipe at it!" I exclaimed.

"Wow, I've never heard of such a thing," Mike said empathetically. "Why would he be so persistent? It's just wrong."

Mike is not much for anger, but I could sense it in his tone. He was put off in the extreme that I had been pestered so frequently by Dr. Hillary.

As the tension slowly subsided and the conversation shifted, Mike remembered the things he had brought from the store for me. He reached inside the bag and pulled out a bottle of organic grape juice and a carton of organic eggs.

"Thank you for getting those," I said as I pointed to a cup sitting by the sink. "There's a cup over there we can mix them in."

Mike stepped to the sink and grabbed the cup. Carefully he cracked two eggs into it. "I'm going to need a fork," he said, as he exited the room.

Two or three minutes later he returned with a plastic fork and began stirring up my concoction. "There you go," he said, pulling a funny face and handing me the cup.

I smiled and chugged it, noting that it was not the most pleasant thing to drink.

That evening as it was getting dark it dawned on me what day it was. "Oh, my gosh," I said turning toward Mike. "It's your birthday."

I sounded much less enthusiastic than I wanted. The medications made every action or verbal expression slow and labored. I sounded old.

He tipped his chin sideways and pulled half a grin. "Yup."

"Whoa. It would have been a really crappy day to die," I said, thinking that the possibility had existed and how difficult it must have been for Mike to realize it.

His smile broadened as he said, "But you didn't."

"I'm sorry," I replied. "I didn't even get you a gift."

He responded quickly, "Yes. Yes you did. You are still alive. That is gift enough."

Then he stood, leaned over me and kissed me, whispering, "You're still here."

~

Sometime around ten o'clock, Mike made another egg cocktail for me, delivering it with a wisecrack, something about chickens getting drunk on grape juice. "It's not fair to make me laugh with brand new stitches," I joked.

Mike sat the cup on the sink then bent, kissing my cheek and whispering, "I love you. Sorry to make you laugh, but that's my job. Sleep tight and happy dreams. I'll see you in the morning. I should be back around nine."

Before Mike even had a chance to gather his things and say good-bye, I nodded off to sleep, not really recognizing that I was even drowsy.

Sometime in the middle of the night I awoke. The glow from the parking lot lights streamed in through my north-facing window. My eyes scanned the room and I wondered what time it was. The hospital seemed very quiet so I estimated that it was likely after midnight.

Immediately to my left, I was unexpectedly aware that an unseen person was present; I felt them gently touch my shoulder. Even though it was dark, I could see well enough to know that no living person was standing there. I briefly questioned it, wondering if it were something else, a muscle spasm or a shift in the fabric of my gown. But then as my awareness increased I felt a sensation that sprang to life and I knew this was something more than earthly. My heart swelled within me as though pyrotechnics had just been ignited there.

As the feeling grew, another invisible hand began touching my other shoulder as I recognized that there were two people in my room. They were there to watch over me and there was an understanding that they had already been doing so filled my heart. That explained my ability to make important decisions even though I was drugged, much to Dr. Hillary's chagrin.

The beings' presence was as tangible as anything I had ever known; I could not see them but I know they were real. Whoever they were, not only was their touch full of love and soothing to me, I was aware that they knew I loved them and appreciated their touch too.

I thought, "I don't know who you are, but I feel you. Thank you."

Many times up to this point, my faith had wavered, but on this particular night, I found myself solid and sure of my imminent recovery. God will not leave you comfortless. He sends help through others. I closed my eyes and felt the love, then fell back to sleep again.

I was awakened one more time, in the wee hours of the morning, by a phlebotomist who had come to draw some blood, then quickly fell back to sleep after she left.

~

The next morning the sun poured over the mountain, sending a bright yellow hue into my window that awoke me. I found it interesting that I felt quite alert and perky, considering everything that had transpired during the night. A nurse came in to check on me, and reminded me to order breakfast. As she was leaving, Mike stepped into the room.

"How nice; you're early!" I said.

"Good morning sunshine," he announced. "You look like you're feeling better, and yes, I'm early ... don't rub it in," he said with a wink.

Mike had never been a morning person, so the fact that he was willing to get out of bed and be there before his appointed hour was impressive.

"I'm glad you came early! I had some visitors last night," I said with enthusiasm.

Mike looked surprised. "Who in the world would show up after I left? What was it, ten?"

"Yes, but they came closer to midnight," I said smirking.

Mike looked perplexed until I began to detail my experience. His eyes became shiny and a tear slipped from the corner, rolling down his cheek. "Wow," he said softly. "I guess the Lord has bigger plans for you. I told you. You're supposed to stay here and live a full life!"

Twenty minutes later, around nine o'clock, Dr. Browning arrived. He announced, "Well, I can't explain it, but you're not anemic anymore."

I smiled. I knew exactly why I was not anemic anymore—grape juice, eggs, and angels. "I don't see any reason to keep you any longer," Dr. Browning said. "You can go home."

Chapter Thirty-Three

THE RECIPIENT OF BLESSINGS

I always knew that angels existed. What I did not grasp, at first, was how frequently they were in my presence, or the fact that they often showed themselves. Sometimes they were completely unseen, like my visitors in the hospital. Other times they came right through my front door to rub my feet or teach me important lessons. Some even wore cowboy hats. They were very real and impacted my life in profound ways that are difficult to express.

When I arrived home the next day, Mike settled me into the downstairs guest bedroom so I would not have to navigate the stairs. Mom and Dad were still there and since I had just taken over their room, they moved into our upstairs bedroom for the night. I felt happy to be home a day or two earlier than expected, due to something as simple as eggs, grape juice, and angels.

My confidence in Don's knowledge, my own intellect about holistic healing, and my steady faith became like granite in my heart—concrete and permanent. There was something satisfying about making the decisions about my own health without the pressure of the medical profession, especially since many of their views ran counter to my own. It became a partnership with Heavenly Father, this faith-driven life I chose, and He taught me each and every day.

On Saturday morning, Mom and Dad packed to leave. It was hard to let them go. I am certain Mom was ready to be in her own home and Dad was ready to have her there.

My mother and I had never had an opportunity to spend time like this since I had grown up and moved out, so our time together, although difficult, was something to be treasured. Our relationship was strengthened and letting her go was bitter sweet.

"I'm going to miss being with you," Mom said as she sat on the couch next to me.

I swallowed hard and held back my own emotions.

She smiled and wrapped me in a gentle embrace. Then she kissed my cheek. We sat there hugging for a long time. I had grown so sensitive to spiritual and emotional things, that I easily felt Mom's love. It entered into my chest and lingered there, long after she had released me.

I smiled as Mom and Dad stepped out the front door. Mike waved to them and then pressed against the doorknob. I felt a little like a child again, not wanting my mother to leave me, but it was time. A wave of grief brushed by me and all of a sudden everything seemed way too quiet. I must have pulled a face because the next thing I knew, Mike was consoling me.

"It's going to be okay, honey," he said, reading my emotions as if I were an open book.

"I know," I said. "In some ways I'm a little scared to be without her; she's been such a rock for me, but mostly I'm just going to miss her." Mike walked over and sat down next to me.

"I get that. It definitely is going to be different, but we'll manage."

"It will seem very strange not to have her here. I'm sure grateful that you will be. I don't know what I would have done without you either," I said in disbelief. "You're amazing."

"I told you I wasn't going anywhere," he said as he took my hand in his.

I smiled. "That's true, you did. But honestly, I don't think there are many men out there who would have stuck it out. This has been a horrible ordeal for you to have to deal with."

"Well, you're worth it," he said as he smiled and pulled me to him into a side embrace.

"I guess we can pretty much make it through anything, can't we?" I said.

"Of course we can; we have each other." I heard a puff of air slip from his nose that told me he had just chuckled, which made me feel secure of his commitment and love for me.

He held me gently for the longest time. It was sweet and quiet and powerful.

Five hours later, Mom texted, "We're home. Miss you already."

"Miss you too! Thank you again for everything you did! I love you so much! Tell Dad thank you for the extended loan. His sacrifice did not go unnoticed," I wrote back.

~

It was Sunday afternoon, two days after I had arrived home and Don called to see how I was doing. I was touched by his generosity and without expectation.

"How are you?" he asked with a smile on his voice.

"It's so good to be home," I said. "The food alone has made me feel so much better! One more day of hospital cuisine and I think I might have keeled over and died."

He chuckled, "You're so funny. I'm so glad you're home. I was so worried about you! Now, what do you say we get you back on your feet?"

"That sounds divine," I responded. "I'm pretty sick and tired of being sick and tired."

As Don spoke, I took note of everything he said. He talked about whole foods, and clean drinking water, and being out in the sunshine. He probably spent about ten minutes detailing what I should be doing to regain my strength. He finished by saying, "You need to get back to walking as soon as possible." And then in that sweet, country twang of his, "I love ya, girl."

"Can I just tell you again how much I love you?" I began. "I don't know of a single person on earth who would have just given of their time and knowledge like you have. When this all started, you really didn't even know me. Thank you so much," I said with great sincerity.

"Aw, you're welcome purty lady." I could almost see him blush.

As we finished our conversation, I hung up the phone with a pretty big smile on my face. I even giggled, grateful for having him as one of my most essential angels.

~

One of the biggest challenges I had yet to face was allowing some of my new circle of four hundred into my home to assist with the things Mom had so efficiently been doing. It was a difficult thing for me to consider. I had never been much for accepting charity, though I was certainly happy to give it. So, when Janice, a lady from church came over and began scheduling meals and women to come and sit with me in three-hour increments, I was annoyed with myself.

Not only had I just gotten out of the worst tribulation of my life, which required more faith than I had ever had to tap into, I realized I had a pride issue as well. It exasperated me.

As Janice sat at the foot of my bed detailing how it would all work, I felt my brow furrow deeply and I began to argue with her—at least in my mind.

"Are you serious?" My beliefs were spinning unrestrained. "Three women a day to clean and cook for me, and then what, are they just supposed to sit here and watch me heal?"

The rosy patches on my neck were beginning to erupt again; I could feel them.

A hundred reasons for not having the ladies come over came to mind. And then reality sunk in; I could not do this without them. Mike would be at work all day and there was no way I could take care of myself just yet. It took all of ten seconds to know I had to do it.

Humbled, I said, "Janice, thank you. I appreciate everything you're offering. Everything you proposed will be fine," I said in surrender.

"Great! Olivia, Karen and Cami will be here tomorrow for their shifts. That should get you within an hour or so of Mike's arrival home from work," she efficiently declared as she jotted something down on her clipboard. I had been beat but I smiled anyway.

The next morning, Mike left early for work. He had used up his entire vacation allotment on this one, difficult situation. There would be no more days off for him until at least the end of August, so there were no options. I selfishly wanted him to stay, but I knew he could not.

"I gotta run, Babe," Mike said as he leaned in and kissed my forehead.

"It's going to be all right," he started. "The time will pass quickly and I'll be home again. You'll see." He smiled at me and turned to leave, "I love you!"

As I sat there in the silence of an empty house, it occurred to me that it had been two months since I had been alone. I was leaning on the headboard of the bed in the spare room with pillows propping me up on both sides. Closing my eyes, I tried to mentally prepare for the changes that were going to happen in a few short minutes when my first caretaker arrived.

There were so many things I could not deny were orchestrated by God— Don, Mom, Mike's vacation availability, Dad coming to the ER, my surgical team, angels, and now the selfless women from church. Heavenly Father knew what I was going to need all along the way.

"If it were all going to happen, it couldn't have happened in a more precise and choreographed way," I silently said. "Thank you Lord, for everything."

After that, it became easier for me to see the Lord's hand in my life, lining up everything in perfect harmony. What had begun as an interruption in my psyche was now another recognition of blessings. Everything was happening for unknown spiritual reasons, and as odd as it sounds, I was the recipient of more blessings than can be measured. I reminded myself that it always works out in the end, even if it's impossible to see sometimes.

Chapter Thirty-Four

THE PERSISTENT DR. HILLARY

That first week after I had arrived home from the hospital, there were many phone calls. Most of them well-wishers calling to send their love for a speedy recovery. But the most striking phone calls came from Dr. Hillary's office, the oncologist I had met in the hospital. For the first four days—in a row—his office called to incessantly solicit for business. It was evident that it was one of Satan's last ditch efforts to knock me off my course.

When I answered the first call a pleasant voice said, "Hello, Mrs. Blickfeldt, this is Dr. Hillary's office. I'm just calling to get you scheduled to come in and see the doctor."

I was surprised and said, "Really? I wasn't planning on coming in, so no thank you."

I was impressed by the doctor's persistence, even shocked. I wondered if our in-hospital conversations were open ended in some way. Our conversations left no doubt in my mind, so I was surprised that Dr. Hillary thought there was some expectation of snagging me as a patient.

The receptionist did not quite know what to say to my rejection. She stammered a bit and eventually thanked me for my time. Then she hung up.

The second call was similar in nature, utilizing a technique I learned in business.

She said, "Dr. Hillary said to tell you your appointment is set for tomorrow morning."

My mouth began forming a severe rebuttal, but I caught myself before letting the words out. It was not this young woman's fault, it was not her agenda … it was Dr. Hillary's.

I took in a breath and began to shut her down before she really knew what hit her. Kindly but firmly I said, "No. Thank you anyway. I won't be coming in tomorrow. Goodbye." At that I hung up the phone without waiting for the customary farewell.

I was increasingly annoyed by the doctor's tenacity, but kept my cool, regardless.

On the third day when the call came, I was hesitant to pick up the phone because by that time, I recognized the phone number, but I did it anyway.

The young woman's voice was soft and gentle, and full of sparkle. She said, "I'm just calling to let you know we have an opening tomorrow at four o'clock if you'd like to take it."

There was an uneasy pause as I looked for the language to express what I was feeling without being offensive. My brow creased and I could feel my skin blistering. I held my breath and tried to remind myself that this unassuming person had no idea how I was feeling and that I had to be cautious about lashing out at her even though I felt like doing just that.

I heard the woman take a breath in. I expect she was about to check if I was still on the line, but I interrupted that possibility by saying, "No. Thank you for calling though," and then I ended the conversation by hanging up rather abruptly.

Just after the lunch hour on the fourth day, my phone rang again. My eyes grew wide and I shook my head in disbelief as I recognized the familiar number. I rolled my eyes and answered.

"Hello?" I said, holding my frustration and keeping my tone emotionless and calm.

"Mrs. Blickfeldt, hi, this is Mia at Dr. Hillary's office. He asked me to give you a call and see if we could get you scheduled to come in on Monday at three?" she said kindly.

I closed my eyes and let the words form. I was careful and considerate of Mia's position in all of this and said, "No, Mia. I'm not coming in. Please tell Dr. Hillary to take me off his list and to never call my home again. Your office has called me for four days in a row and each time I have said no. I actually mean it. I'm not coming in to see him. In fact, if I ever were to see an oncologist it would never be him!"

My voice was measured and hard, and I think Mia was a bit shocked at my strong declaration because the line was uncomfortably silent for at least ten seconds.

Then she spoke. "Uh … Oh, um, okay. Well, uh, thank you then," she said stammering over herself as if she had tripped over a log. "I, uh, I'm so sorry to disturb you."

"It's all right, just please pass my message on to Dr. Hillary," I stated flatly.

"I will be sure to do that," she said. "Thank you. Good bye."

And that was the end of the persistent Dr. Hillary. I had to give him credit, though—and an "e" for effort, an "e" for his relentless, incessant efforts. I was not about to budge from my plan of holistic healing, which had obviously worked, to move on to his plan of chemotherapy … which I had zero faith in. That would be ludicrous.

~

Don called again a week later. "How ya doin' girl?" he asked in his usual cowboy voice.

"So much better. The last seven days I've had nothing but help, but I've recovered so quickly that I'm up and moving around the house by myself now," I reported proudly.

"Well then, suck it up girl and get moving! Air, sunshine, and walking is the key to your healing and recovery. Now get out there! Start with five minutes, and then move up to twenty, then eventually an hour. It's just one foot in front of the other." He made it sound so easy.

I put on my shoes and stepped outside. I was pretty wobbly and felt embarrassed at my appearance. I had lost a lot of weight, so all the clothes I wore hung loosely on my bones and appeared more like a scary Halloween costume. My hair was abnormally untidy and pulled back on both sides away from my face, making me look even more skeletal.

"You win, Don," I said as I turned my face to the sun. It felt good to be outside. "Dang it! Why do you always have to be right?" The words slipped from my lips with a little more annoyance than they should have, and then I snickered to myself.

I stood still in the light of the afternoon for a few minutes, just letting it soak in. I felt happy and fresh . . . and alive! I filled my lungs. They hurt a little as I forced as much air in as possible, but it was a glorious discomfort. It was like my body was sparking with life.

Turning, I began plodding slowly up the sidewalk. My muscles screamed in pain, and delight. All I could do was laugh. I doubt I even made it twenty-five yards before I knew I was spent and had to turn around. It was not much but at least it was a start.

After that day, I made it a daily practice to get outside and walk. I made it further and further every day, until one day I realized I had made it all the way around the path.

In ceremonious style, I carefully and gently jumped up and down with my clenched hands above my head as though I were an athlete who had just won an Olympic gold medal. I knew then that I was well on my way to getting back to living.

~

As the weeks wore on, I grew stronger and stronger, with my muscles rebuilt to where I could easily walk for an hour. Every cell in my body was enlivened and I knew that Heavenly Father had delivered me from the grips of death. He had fulfilled his promises. It was not exactly the way I had anticipated the process to go but, nonetheless, I was healed.

Sometimes I still wonder what would have happened if I had confronted the *procedure* early on in my journey. I would have become a different person than I am now, and I would have missed everything. As peculiar as it sounds, that would have been a tragedy. There was entirely too much gained to spend even one second imagining my experiences any differently.

Now that it is behind me, I can easily say that I am changed for the better forever. I have come to know, unequivocally, that when you nurture the seeds that you plant, your roots grow deep into the earth of your own truth; and when you truly believe … anything is possible.

Chapter Thirty-Five

NEW LIFE

After my surgery, it took about two months to re-engage in life and begin planning my music career in earnest. I was ready to live like I had never lived before—full on! I sensed a powerful self-assuredness that had not existed prior to having cancer, and I knew that I was about to crack my musical aspirations wide open and create everything I had envisioned for myself. As soon as the cobwebs cleared from my brain, I could clearly see that *becoming* was as simple as an attitude change. I could be whatever I imagined.

A musical plan developed as I began filling my calendar, scheduling those who could help me progress and fulfill my musical aspirations. In turn, I was eager to help them reach theirs, too.

As I met with a few very connected individuals, I quickly began to see where my ideas would fit into the highly competitive music industry.

One afternoon I met with an internationally recognized composer, vocal performer, and recording artist, Paul Cactus Jack La Marr. We sat down at a small outdoor table in a quaint shopping area. I was a bit nervous because, in reality, I had no clue how to get from point A to point B. I had completely embraced the concept of just going for it, so I jumped in with both feet by asking, "Where is it that you hope to take your career?"

His response took me a bit off guard, but as soon as he said it, I knew I had found a good mentor. He said, "All the way."

He knew exactly what he wanted and where he was going. A few minutes later he asked me, "Did you bring any recordings with you?"

I had. I was eager and nervous for him to listen. As he placed the earphones to his ears, he leaned forward placing his elbows onto his knees. I instinctively drew in a long deep breath and held it. From my angle, all I could see was the top of his head. It made me nervous. I could not see his eyes. My palms began to sweat and I felt my heart flutter and begin to pound out a beat of its own. In my mind a million thoughts began swirling in.

Cactus had no way of knowing, but I admired him. His accomplishments were at a point that I recognized how important his recommendations could be to me. This moment would either make or break me. His word would mean more than anyone I had spoken to yet. He likely had no idea that I felt this way, but he had great influence over my uncertain and tenuous ambitions. It crossed my mind that after everything I had been through, that stubborn part of me was surprisingly willing to trust someone outside of my circle, even if it was for an entirely different reason. But I did. And for me, this was the moment of truth.

I wiped my palms across the thigh of my jeans, leaving them there and hoping they would not look as wet as they felt. My heart beat a little louder as my blood pressure rose another level. As I stared at the top of Cactus' head, all I could see were a few unsettling head shakes.

He listened for a while and then he lifted his head a little and stated in a rather disturbing tone, "Finally!" He glanced up, catching my eye. There was a critical glint in his. "I was wondering when it would stop sounding like karaoke." He dropped his head back down.

An imaginary blade the size of a bowie knife plunged into my heart and it stopped beating for a moment, suspended temporarily in terror. Everything around me seemed to stop. I had already been frozen in place, but now I was completely rigid. My muscles began to shake. "He hates me!" I thought for several seconds, my eyes glassing over. And then like a kettle drum, my heart restarted, banging violently against the inner wall of my body. I could feel the blood rush back to my cheeks.

I closed my eyes and let his words sear into me, "Maybe I'm just not ready for this. Maybe I'm just not that good." Every inch of my skin pulsated in defeat and I bowed my head, feeling as though I might cry. The weight of my imaginings were growing with each passing second, and sweat beaded up on the hairline at the top of my forehead.

I could barely detect the sound from the mp3 player, but I could see that Cactus was cutting a few of the songs short and moving on to the next without listening to them in their entirety. "He hates me. That's it. I'm done before I even get started." My stomach was turning in knots. Tension built within me as I envisioned my dreams evaporating right before me. I swallowed hard, mostly to stop the ache from inching its way up. I was not going to cry! I was pretty sure that he was completely disappointed with me. He kept shaking his head back and forth, and so did I as I mirrored his actions. It just fed the fire of defeat even more profoundly.

I noted that he turned the volume up and suddenly I could hear which song he was listening to. A minute or two into the music, Cactus lifted his chin from where it was resting on his hands and stared up at me with an absorbed look. "This could be your signature song," he said, dropping his chin and closing his eyes again.

My head spun, "What?" I voiced inside myself. "What did you say? 'Signature' … does that mean you like it?" I immediately sat up straight and the heaviness lifted from off my shoulders and floated far away. My emotions turned from their previously infused grey space, into light. It was so quick that I could barely allow myself to believe what I was thinking. I held my breath, watching intently like a predatory animal ready to pounce.

Then I watched as Cactus clicked to the last song on the playlist. I took a breath in and held it again. *This* was the song I was most anxious for him to listen to, because I thought it was really well done. If he liked it, then there might be a chance. Did I even dare hope?

Working to regain my composure, I began praying a childish prayer, "Oh please, oh please, oh please let him like it; let him like it, please, please." Completely focused on his every move, every facial expression, every cue from his body language, he shook his head again. My heart banged against my ribs causing not a little pain. "Was that a good headshaking or a bad one?" I tried to surmise as the beads of sweat beginning to roll down. I reached up and wiped it, wondering what his thoughts were.

My anxiety was mounting as I clearly heard the crescendo of the music rise higher and higher. If I had been a soap bubble, I might have just popped. "Here we go," I said out loud, unintentionally as I heard my voice rising higher with the music.

Cactus heard me speak and lifted his eyes. I flinched my head backward in near panic that I had interrupted him. He looked at me dead on, his eyes were red and bloodshot, and brimming with tears. He said nothing but let his head fall back down toward the ground.

My mouth might have dropped open at that point. I am not entirely certain, but I was sure that shock registered on my face. I was glad he was not looking at me just then. "He likes it?" I whispered quietly so as not to disturb him again.

A sliver of hope slipped into my mind and started filling me with a warm glow and I instinctively smiled, "He likes it; I think he likes it," I questioned silently as I began another conversation with myself.

Generally, a gauge of my success in any given performance was when I noticed someone crying. That meant they were spiritually touched. But this was completely unexpected! Cactus was a professional, after all, who was here to be critical of my gift, not moved by it. As that realization settled over me, my smile grew a little larger.

The song concluded and Cactus removed the ear phones. I quickly wiped the smile from my face so that he would not see it. I had to be composed and poised. For a moment he just stared at me, saying nothing. It was like sitting on pins and needles as I waited for his thoughts. I may have winced a bit. His emotion was real and I could sense it. A tear streaked down his cheek. He reached up, wiping it with his finger, and then he spoke, "Wow," was all he said and then he shook his head again.

I had nothing to say, I just stared back letting reality seep into every cell of my body, pervading me with joy. He drew in a breath and began talking about my talent and where I could take it. How impressed he was with my overall look and demeanor, my desire to succeed. Every previous uncertainty instantaneously cleared and I was transported to a place of absolute confidence and surety.

As I drove home that day, all I could do was giggle. It seemed that everything was finally beginning to line up! I could hardly believe it. I literally reached over and pinched myself to see if it was real. It was… very real.

And then life happened.

Again.

Chapter Thirty-Six

YOU JUST CAN'T MAKE THIS STUFF UP!

About a month after, late on a chilly summer evening just after dark, three of my friends and I pulled into the parking lot at Wasatch Mountain State Park in Midway, Utah. We had been on a lengthy horseback ride to the top of the mountains. It was August 11, just over five months since my cancer surgery.

Danica was there, laughing and telling silly jokes; my friend Shelly, whom I had just reconnected with after a number of years; and Jeremy—he was driving. He was the epitome of a western cowboy. From his boots to his chaps to his hat, he was the real deal. He was chuckling to himself as he pressed on the brake bringing the truck to a halt. Then he switched on the interior cab light, wiggled the gear shift and set the parking brake.

Everyone reached to open their doors, except Shelly, who was collecting her personal items into her arms.

Momentarily, I hesitated, not knowing why, but it struck me that I did it. I glanced over my left shoulder and noticed that Danica had opened her door, gathered her things and moved to get out. Jeremy had shifted his weight and leaned low so his hat would not hit the door jamb as he exited.

I turned back to my already open door wondering why I hesitated. I had my cell phone in one hand and a digital camera in the other. I began sliding off of the seat to the ground, which was a few inches below where I could reach. It was very dark and I could not see the blacktop. Then something strange happened. Instantly I sensed movement. It was as though the ground itself was moving, like someone had grabbed a rug and yanked it out from underneath me.

Immediately I had the sense of falling. It was quite surreal and in very slow motion. One of those moments when you realize that your thoughts are moving faster than your brain. "Oh dang it!" I thought to myself. "I'm falling and my hands are full! I won't be able to break my fall."

And then I landed . . . hard! Both hands hit the ground first, smashing my camera and phone into the asphalt. Frustrated ideas came fast and with full force, "Oh no, my camera! I'll never be able to afford to replace it! The lens alone is worth five hundred dollars! Oh, I hope I didn't shatter my phone! I've never broken a phone, I wonder if my contract is up yet. I hope I don't have to replace it. Cell phones are so expensive!" Annoyance draped over me at the idea of having to replace my equipment.

So many thoughts passed through my mind. I barely had time to adjust to the fact that I had fallen. That sense was immediately substituted by the realization that I had fallen onto the right side of my body and my head had just slammed into the ground. "Ooof," the noise bolted from my mouth as the air forced its way out of me. I groaned and began to formulate a thought about getting up.

Abruptly, a different and sudden comprehension struck me. The bottom of my boot was caught beneath something. "The tire? It's the tire!" I screamed to myself. The rolling front tire of Jeremy's six-ton pickup was on my boot! "What the heck? What's happening? Is my foot getting run over? The truck is rolling! But I saw him put the brake on! It's just the heel of my boot. Is it just the heel? Will it hold the weight? What if it crushes the heel? Surely it'll be off in a second and then I can get up." Before I could even process any of those fleeting ideas and react, something else happened.

Just behind my left leg I felt the tire grab ahold of me at the hip as it began climbing up my backside. I screamed, realizing that I was in serious trouble.

In a very involuntary fashion, shrieks filled the air, dashing the silence of the night. It barely entered my thoughts that it was me.

Every dark and negative idea that could have come to me was now being acted out in frantic, chaotic, deadly disorder. I imagined Mike kneeling and crying at my graveside, my children grief-stricken at losing their mother, the shock on my friend's faces as they realized I had been killed. Everything that really mattered in life was suddenly thrust into the forefront and a great sadness moved in like a gloomy shadow on a drizzly day. I thought of my budding music career and the unsung songs that would never pass over my lips, and the people I would never impact.

My screams seemed to last forever, hitting my ears with piercing tones of sheer terror. They faded in and out as if someone were turning the knob on a stereo up and then down and then up again, rattling my senses with their vibrations. I wanted to make it stop.

I wanted to move away from the images that were bombarding me—my smashed body lying motionless underneath that tire, blood oozing from the injuries, blank eyes staring into the starry sky. My mind spun wildly, seeing the final outcome of my situation and terror gripped me like some kind of Halloween specter with boney fingers.

"I can't die now!" The words pressed sharply against my forehead. "Not now! I just got healed! I can't die this way! No!" All this passed through my mind as screams sounded.

Milliseconds later, as the truck continued its slow-motion climb up the back of my hip, it reached the back edge of my belt. Miracles of miracles, the leather strapping that was attached to metal loops that held my belt together suddenly broke beneath the crushing weight. The tires bounced just behind me, setting me free from the mighty jaws that held me bound.

Instinct kicked in and straightaway I rolled twice, away from the truck. When I came to a stop, I found myself lying on my left side in a patch of freshly mowed grass that lay right next to the blacktop. My heart shuddered and thumped violently beneath my skin. "I'm alive," I heard myself whisper.

I tried to put together a cohesive thought about what had just happened and what I should be doing about it. Pain shot through my hips. I squeezed my eyes shut and let out a deep sounding growl that climbed up from the middle of my core and shot from my mouth. I was feeling excruciating pain.

Immediately I began silently praying, "Heavenly Father," I screamed within, "I'm in trouble! If there is anything broken, or out of place in my body, could you please put it back and minimize the damage as much as possible. Please, please, please?"

The agony began to mount; twisting around my hip like someone had placed it in a clamp and tightened it until I thought I would blackout. Sparking flashes of glittery stars danced before my eyes. I blinked hard and breathed shallowly, trying not to hyperventilate. Then I lifted my eyes and watched as the truck jerked to a halt, the tires skidding against the pavement.

"Wait," I thought, "Jeremy is back in the truck. He's just now stopping it." I watched as the truck came to a complete stop. "Why did it take so long? So much has happened since I fell." I thought ... and then I understood.

In a flash I knew what many others had described; time was tangled. I was sure it had been at least two minutes since I had fallen; however, in reality, it had only been a few seconds—just long enough for Jeremy to get out of the truck and realize it was rolling.

"The headlights are on, they were off before or it wouldn't have been so dark," I deliberated. "I can hear Danica's voice, where is she? Where's Shelly? Is she still in the truck?" Then I saw her feet reaching the ground from where she had been sitting in the backseat. Then I saw all of their feet running in my direction.

Laying there, I intuitively knew not to move. I pushed my right hand onto the blacktop to stabilize my body, which lay just at the edge of the grassy area. I attempted to move the pebbles that were cutting my palm by shifting the weight onto my hips momentarily so I could brush them aside. Pain ripped through me and I screamed again. I could not brush them aside. It was imperative that I not move.

Intentionally I slowed my breathing; it was irregular as my heartbeat, which was beating erratically against my sides. "You have to keep the pressure off," I said without speaking. Slowly, I pushed up with my hand, onto my fingertips, keeping the pressure balanced. Carefully I swiped my thumb underneath struggling to dislodge the rocks that were digging into my hand and deliberately working to not move my lower body. The rocks rolled from beneath my palm so I pressed it flat trying to lift even more pressure off of myself. Whatever had just happened inside of me, I knew the damage was in my hips and most likely in my foot, too. I could feel blood trickling down my forehead.

"Heavenly Father, thank you for helping me to move away from the truck," I began my silent prayer, "Please, help me to get through this, and please bless my body to heal from whatever damage has been done."

Pushing all the weight I could onto my right hand, I began adjusting my left one, which had been lying just in front of my face. Slowly and methodically, I moved it to where it created a cushion between the grass and my head, blood quickly spilling through my fingers and into the grass. The ball cap I had been holding was still hooked around my pinky finger.

Noises began to fill my ears as I heard Jeremy and Danica's voices, becoming louder as they came running around the front of the truck and over to where I was.

Jeremy's voice elevated to a higher pitch than was usual for him. As he reached me he fell to one knee just in front of my legs. "Alicia! Oh my hell! Alicia! Alicia! Are you okay? What can I do to help?" His tone was fiercely desperate. I could hear his breathing, short, fast, and heavy. He was panicked.

My first thought was that I needed a blessing and proceeded to ask him for one. "Jeremy, give me a blessing!" I demanded as forcefully as I could, but it sounded more like a murmur. Danica was talking fast and loud, but I could not make out her words. Shelly cried out, "Oh my heck! What do we do?"

Jeremy did not respond to my plea. In all the upheaval I expect he simply did not hear me so I tried again, "Jeremy … give me a blessing right now." It came out a little louder but still it did not get his attention. I could see him looking around, thrashing his arms up and down, and talking at Shelly. Then he turned to Danica. His eyes were wide and filled with terror. Then he placed both hands on either side of his face and shook it back and forth.

Drawing in as big a breath as I could, I spoke again, "Jeremy, give me a blessing, right now! Right now! I need a blessing now!" I used up every last ounce of air I had taken in; my voice still not much louder than a librarian.

Jeremy looked at me as the words finally registered to him. He stared a little harder.

"Jeremy, I need a blessing! Give me a blessing, now!" I said again, as loud as I could.

His expression spoke volumes. He looked decidedly hesitant. Instinctively I knew that he did not feel capable of the task I was requesting of him. His jaw dropped open and I watched as he reached up and put his forehead into the palm of his hand.

He breathed deeply, dropped his other knee and crept closer, accepting the task I had just presented him. He looked humbled and broken, and unsure of himself. He shook his head again and then turned, asking Danica and Shelly if they knew my full name.

It is customary to address a person by their full name and I knew that Jeremy did not know mine. He was of course familiar with my first and last name, but not my middle name. In his shock, he neglected to hear me verbalize it. Then

I said, "I know my name, Jeremy." But he just did not hear me. I said my name three or four times, but he was not listening.

I drew in another deep breath, as deep as I could anyway and said, "Jeremy," the voice did not sound like mine and was louder than I had the capacity to exert, "I know my name."

The atmosphere changed and the gravity of my request brought a solemnity that none of us expected. A hush fell over the others as Jeremy reached up and took off his cowboy hat and laid it on the ground next to his left knee.

The first miracle happened when Jeremy reached over and placed his hands on my head. I closed my eyes and before a word had even been spoken, the pain began to disperse. It softened to a level that was curiously tolerable.

I heard very few of the words from the blessing, with the exception of the phrase, "Everything is going to be fine."

That was all I needed to hear. My heart slowed as I repeated it internally multiple times, "Everything is going to be fine. Everything is going to be fine."

When my faith had been taken to the very limit with my cancer, I had learned to trust God, so I was not about to question what I had come to trust so implicitly. I just knew that what Jeremy had spoken was a direct statement from Heavenly Father to me.

Jeremy removed his hands. I opened my eyes and caught sight of Danica who was standing close. "Danica, please call for help," I pleaded. It struck me that I was the one suggesting it. By the look on her face she was still in shock, and it took her a second to understand my request. She glanced down at her phone and dialed a number. I heard her repeat the details of the accident and request an ambulance.

When she ended the call, I moaned, "Please call Mike." It came out more like someone with a speaking disorder, short, halted and broken. Breathing hurt.

"Your phone is shattered and I don't have his number," she said with an alarmed pitch.

"I know it," I breathed out, grateful that I was conscious and able to give her the number.

"Yes, she's conscious and talking with us," I heard her say as she recounted what happened to Mike. "We're not really sure what's wrong; the ambulance is on its way. I'll call you as soon as I know anything."

"What? What do you mean you'll call him as soon as you know anything? He needs to be here now! Why didn't you tell him to come now? I need him!" My mind was in commotion.

Then I heard her say, "Yes. Yes. Okay." And then she hung up the phone.

While we waited for the ambulance, I brooded over the phone call to Mike. I wanted to tell her to call him back, but I was growing weaker by the moment and all my concentration needed to be focused on holding my bodyweight still. I lamented internally, "Was he really not coming yet?" I silently cried a tearless cry and suffocated in my own heartache.

After a time I reconnected with the conversation and listened to the others discuss what happened as if I were not there. It struck me as odd. They were all standing a few paces away and the sound of their voices twirled through the air in subdued, hollow tones. I felt a little non-existent. I wanted to join the discussion, but there was no energy to be expended for that.

Jeremy said, "I don't know what happened. I put the brake on just like I always do."

Danica put a hand on his shoulder. "It was an accident," she said, trying to comfort him.

"Tell that to Alicia," he said loudly, pointing his thumb in my direction.

"Oh Jeremy, it was an accident. You know that," Shelly commented with compassion.

"Of course it was," I said to myself. I wished I could tell him right then.

Feeling weary, I disengaged from their comments and turned inward again, wondering why this would happen. Why was this happening now? Things were just starting to pop in my life. I thought about the possible extent of the damage to my body, and I speculated as to how long it would take to recover from the injuries. I knew I would recover, Jeremy's blessing stated that clearly, but that did not stop me from questioning the logistics of the situation.

I felt calm, but frozen in place when several sheriffs' vehicles arrived. I was growing tired of holding my body in such an abnormal position and my arm began to shake.

One of the officers bent over, asking my name and where I lived, and when my birthday was. He was simply assessing me, especially since he could easily see the cut on my temple. In some ways it was a welcome distraction from what I had been thinking.

An ambulance arrived with several EMTs. I screamed as they placed a brace around my neck. They slid a gurney underneath my body. I screamed again and then they wheeled me into the back of the ambulance.

After arriving at the hospital, I was taken into the emergency room and evaluated, x-rayed and scanned. A momentary annoyance filled me as I thought about what Don would say to that. But I knew in this case, they had to be taken. They gave me some pretty heavy-duty medication that took away the pain. Even in my self-adopted, holistic lifestyle, I was glad for the relief.

When I began to feel more comfortable, Jeremy, Danica, and Shelly were allowed in to see me. Danica announced that Mike was on his way. Seconds later I heard his voice. Just like the many months before after coming out of surgery, it was his voice that brought me comfort.

He had obviously just gotten into the truck and begun driving without asking for updates. Tears sprang to my eyes, and dropped gently onto the sheet near my ears. As he lifted my hands to his, I quickly and quietly thanked God for bringing him safely to my side. Again.

The doctor came in and announced that they did not really have the staff or equipment necessary to handle my other injuries so they were going to transport me to Salt Lake.

Jeremy walked back over to me and touched my hand gently. "Alicia, I am so sorry," he said repeatedly.

"I know Jeremy. It was an accident," I responded compassionately.

And then Jeremy began to cry. His head fell forward into his hand but he did not let go of me with the other. I could literally feel his ache swelling in my body and realized how horrific it must be to feel responsible for another person's injuries.

Strangely, a sense of profound coherency came over me and I said, "Jeremy, someone has already paid for this. Why don't you go home and give it to Him."

Jeremy's chin came up abruptly as his eyes locked with mine. I watched, as what I had said sank in. First shock, and then almost immediately after that, as the words permeated his soul, peace. Christ already paid the price—not only for what I was suffering—but for what Jeremy was suffering, too. Comprehension filled his eyes and he nodded in recognition.

In his soft country twang, Jeremy whispered, "Oh … wow. You're right. I can't believe you. I'm the last person you should be thinking of right now," he said, choking up again, "I can't believe you'd say that. I'm the one who should be consoling you." He squeezed my hand again, just before he turned to leave.

Miracle number two—the Lord had used me to help Jeremy heal from a horrific situation. He needed comfort just as much as I did. The lesson for me was that God will let you be the conduit for others; no matter what you happen to be dealing with, if you are open to it.

Not more than ten minutes later, I was placed in the ambulance and transported to the Salt Lake valley.

~

Mike was sitting in a chair to my left in the room they had placed me in and said, "It's seven a.m. It's been a long night."

"Very," I responded, as I grasped the fact that I had been awake for twenty-four hours. My body had been highly medicated so I was relatively comfortable. Allowing my mind to follow suit, I closed my eyes and quickly fell asleep.

A little over an hour later, a doctor came in, introducing himself as Dr. Corbett. He was tall and nice looking, with blue eyes and glasses. He had a kind, genuine smile and seemed very friendly. It surprised me a little after my previous encounters with some of the doctors earlier in the year.

He stepped to a computer in the corner of the room and began looking at my x-rays and CAT scan, explaining my injuries in detail as he pointed to the screen with his finger. He said that I had a small broken bone in my right foot, and that it was not displaced too far from its original location. He also said there was a break in the orbital bone at the back of my pelvis and several cracks in my pelvic region, including one in the hip socket.

As he spoke, I zoned out as I realized that this was miracle number three. These were my *only* injuries. There should have been more. I wondered how the injuries were not worse.

I flashed back to the accident. Maybe He had answered my prayer right there on the spot while I lay in the grass. Maybe angels were there, gently pulling me away from the tire and the potentialities. I seriously doubt I would have gotten off so lucky if my belt had not broken, which I certainly counted as a blessing. Maybe God had moved my bones into a better position as I had requested. I did not know for sure, but I decided to accept it as another miracle. That was 4.

My thoughts were interrupted by Dr. Corbett's next comment. "We'd like to go in surgically and place a plate and some screws to stabilize the injuries," he stated.

"Will the bones heal without surgery?" I queried.

He looked up at me, studying my eyes and seeming somewhat surprised that I would even ask. "Yes," he said, "I believe they would."

"Then I'm not doing it," I said firmly.

He glanced at the floor, and then he looked back at me. I saw the change in his demeanor as he grasped that I was not budging. He knew he had told me that I would heal regardless, but that did not stop him from trying one last time to convince me that surgery was the best choice.

"You'll heal faster if you agree to the procedures," he said somewhat less firmly than one might anticipate.

My defenses kicked up and I felt the hair on my neck stand up.

I breathed in and then out, "I appreciate that, but no. I think I'll just heal," I said.

He did not press me any further and then said, giving in, "Okay, I'll let you get some rest then. I'll be back tomorrow to check on you." And at that he left the room.

I chuckled within and said, "Well that was easy."

Miracle number five—a complete reliance on God. Suddenly I was grateful for my earlier experiences that helped me make clean and clear decisions now. It was the right decision; I knew it.

~

My expectation of the road that lay before me was that it was going to be difficult. But it did not take much time for me to come to the conclusion that after everything else I had been through that year, healing from the truck accident was going to be a piece of cake.

I spent a full week in the hospital. On the third day there, I was looking through my email when my heart pounded excitedly as I noticed the sender, Utah Music Awards. In some ways it terrified me to open it, but that only lasted a few minutes. I clicked on the link, it read: *"We are pleased to inform you that you have been selected as a nominee for the Utah Music Awards."*

I laughed out loud, loud enough that people in the hallway certainly heard it. A plan began to formulate. It was only eight weeks away and it did not matter if I were walking or not—I was going!

After leaving the hospital, there were three more weeks in a transitional rehabilitation facility, lots of physical therapy, a hospital bed in my living room, and a wheelchair. I had not fixed my hair or worn makeup since the accident, so I was a bit worse for the wear I thought, but the day I rolled into the music awards in my short black, beaded gown, I was elated. I did not care how my hair looked. I was there and I had reached the goal!

EPILOGUE

FOLLOW YOUR HEART

In the end, and as I look back on everything that happened that year, I could never count all of the miracles; they happened every day. I could have died, but I did not. It is obvious *they were wrong* in their declarations about that. Men can never decide when it is your time to progress from this earthly journey—only God can.

I learned, and have come to firmly believe, that everything, especially the hard things in life, have purpose and meaning. My experiences were some of the worst in my life ... and the best. I am different because of them; I am better—and all because I chose to heed the counsel to *follow your heart*. It was a conscious and determined choice that I have come to embrace.

The human body is an amazing thing. I have complete knowledge that it has the ability to heal itself—with the help of the Lord, of course. I know this; it is no longer a question to struggle over. And since I did not die, I intend to live. My path is clear before me. My mission is to fill the world with light—His light—through music. I will not only speak it into reality, I will make it happen. For when God is on your side, you are unconquerable. I am a conqueror.

May you, too, find the path you are meant to take.

CHOICE

Inside my soul there is a space
Where peace replaced the fear.
Overcoming unseen oppression—
A grasp that held me there.

I learned from ache a greater lesson
The other never gleans,
The past is meant to pass on through,
I found another means.

The path I chose was mine to take
Of courage, bright and true.
It showed the way in darkest night,
The road of very few.

There was no force on Earth nor Hell
With strength to take apart.
His gift to me, you know it well,
To follow this, my heart.

What I may leave may seem quite small
But hope you may acquire,
The greatest prize is freely given—
His love will take you higher.

THE END

To follow Alicia's career, look for her on

...

Facebook

Reverbnation

Twitter

SoundCloud

Instagram

&

On YouTube, you will find an artistic interpretation of the journey described in

this book. It is called,

Pie Jesu, The Process of Redemption

#fillingtheworldwithlight

BE OPEN. LISTEN. ACT.

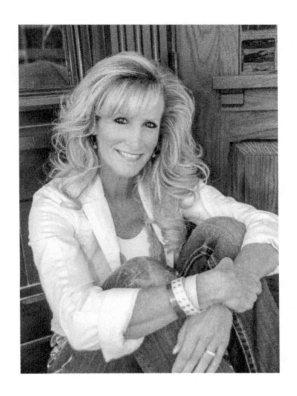

ABOUT ALICIA BLICKFELDT

Firstly, I am not a writer; I am a singer—and that is my passion. But this story was one that needed to be told, so for the first time in my life, I put on the hat of an author … and here we are. I hope it goes over well.

I was born in Ogden, Utah; moved to Pocatello, Idaho when I was nine years old; and then, after spending time in Missouri, Arkansas and Arizona, finally came home to the glorious mountains of Northern Utah— where I intend to stay. It is a perfect fit for me. For as long as I can remember, warm summer evenings were spent at "the cabin," in Huntsville, Utah, which belonged to my grandparents. I am ruined now; city life completely suffocates me. I tried it once or twice.

Throughout high school I participated in every musical event possible. It was about that time I met the now famous opera singer Hans Gregory Ashbaker. I took voice lessons from him for one short summer, but it set me on a path that I have yet to wander away from. Later, I was privileged to take lessons, again, from Weber State University professor Karen Brookens Bruestle for about another four months. I make mention of these brief experiences simply because my voice is purely a gift from God. All that I have created, accomplished, and become is due to Him.

By nature, I am a poet—and a lyricist. My first exposure to singing publically was in church. At age 12 I was asked to participate in a quartet—I did not even know what that meant at the time, but I did it, and I loved it. I sang in every school choir and show I could, but never pursued singing as a career until 2013—the year before I was diagnosed with cancer. It only slowed me down; it certainly did not conquer my spirit.

I am happily and gratefully married to Mike, who has stood unwaveringly by my side through everything imaginable. And to his credit, he is still here, ever blessing my world. He is unbelievably supportive in my musical ventures, encouraging me every single day. My dad always said, "Marry a man who makes you laugh every day." Dad, I did, and you were right. Between Mike and me, we have five living children (there is a story there for another day).

My hobbies include singing, hiking, serving others, photography, and writing poetry, reading, dreaming big and watching those dreams come into fruition. I love God. I love Jesus Christ. I would be nothing without them. I love people, especially those who are working to make a difference in the world, which is a huge part of living life to its fullest.

Recently I was able to compile a team of incredibly talented and giving people who helped me produce a selection of music videos—but stay tuned, there are many more to come!

Alicia Blickfeldt can be reached via email:

aliciablickfeldt@gmail.com